Sex
Made Easy

Your awkward questions answered—
for better, smarter,
Amazing sex

By Debby Herbenick, Ph.D., M.P.H.

Running Press
Philadelphia • London

© 2012 by Debby Herbenick
Published by Running Press,
A member of the Perseus Books Group

All rights reserved under the Pan-American and International Copyright Conventions
Printed in the United States

*This book may not be reproduced in whole or in part, in any form or by any means, electronic or mechanical,
including photocopying, recording, or by any information storage and retrieval system now known or here-
after invented, without written permission from the publisher.*

Books published by Running Press are available at special discounts for bulk purchases in the United States
by corporations, institutions, and other organizations. For more information, please contact the Special
Markets Department at the Perseus Books Group, 2300 Chestnut Street, Suite 200, Philadelphia, PA 19103, or
call (800) 810-4145, ext. 5000, or e-mail special.markets@perseusbooks.com.

ISBN 978-0-7624-4406-9
Library of Congress Control Number: 2011944640

E-book ISBN 978-0-7624-4496-0

9 8 7 6 5 4 3 2 1
Digit on the right indicates the number of this printing

Cover and interior design by Bill Jones

Interior illustrations by Josie Morway

Author photograph © Bernard Gordillo

Edited by Jennifer Kasius
Typography: Conduit, Minion, and French Script

Running Press Book Publishers
2300 Chestnut Street
Philadelphia, PA 19103-4371

Visit us on the web!
www.runningpress.com

This book is dedicated to all of the parents, best friends, partners, school teachers, nurses, doctors, journalists, sex educators, counselors, therapists, activists, spiritual leaders, and politicians who are trying in earnest and with heart to make people's sex lives easier and more enjoyable.

Contents

Acknowledgments

Aiding me in my efforts to make sex a little, if not a lot, easier for readers of this book, a number of people have made my work significantly easier and more pleasant. I am grateful to my editor, Jennifer Kasius, for her patience, direction, and vision and the thoughtful ways in which she helped me to articulate my message. I am thankful to my literary agent, Kate Lee, for believing in my work and for her encouragement and wisdom. The talented Josie Morway deserves praise for gracing these pages with her beautiful illustrations.

Many thousands of women and men inspired this book by trusting me with their sex-related secrets and questions. A number of these are readers of my sex columns and listeners of our *Kinsey Confidential* podcast series whom I have never met. However, not a day goes by that I don't hear from or think about them and the kinds of information that might make their sexual lives easier or more meaningful. Then there are the many women and men whom I've met, or taught at Indiana University, or who have sat in my office—and sometimes cried in my office—as they asked questions and sometimes shared their sexual difficulties with me. This is a kind of trust and intimacy that no schooling could have ever prepared me for and I am grateful to experience it so regularly. It inspires me to want to learn more, research the right questions, and share the answers I find with the people who need them.

I am fortunate, too, to work with a number of colleagues who have provided support, encouragement, laughter—and intellectual stimulation throughout the process of writing—as well as through my day-to-day work of conducting research and teaching about human sexuality. I count myself very lucky to work on a daily basis with Michael Reece, Vanessa Schick, and Brian Dodge; I hope never to take for granted their friendship and camaraderie. I am also indebted to our team of graduate students at the Center for Sexual Health Promotion at Indiana University (Alexis, Andreia, Caroline, Erika, Kristen, Margo, Nicole, Phil, Randy, and Sofia), all of whom

I'm confident will make the world a better place through their research and education efforts. Jennifer Bass, John Bancroft, Thomas Nord, and Jim Lenahan were among the first to put me in charge of answering readers' sex questions and I'm thankful that they believed in me. Additionally, many colleagues, mentors, and former students—whether they know it or not—have inspired and challenged my thinking in ways that I hope have made *Sex Made Easy* a more helpful book. These include Justin Anderson, Michael Bailey, Jada Barbry, Cara Berg, Lee Belz, Virginia Braun, Laura Castiglione, Meredith Chivers, Meredith Davis, Betty Dodson, Christopher Fisher, Dennis Fortenberry, Cindy Graham, Madeline Haller, Julia Heiman, Ariane Hollub, Jordan Humphrey, Natalie Ingraham, Catherine Johnson-Roehr, Jeana Jorgensen, Kristen Jozkowski, Holly Moyseenko Kossover, Wendy Likes, Kate McCombs, Carol McCord, Cindy Meston, Robin Milhausen, Charlene Muehlenhard, Brian Mustanski, Emily Nagoski, Lucia O'Sullivan, Carol Queen, June Reinisch, Heather Rupp, Tracy Rupp, Stephanie Sanders, Sonya Satinsky, Dan Savage, Michaela Schwartz, Samantha Seeger, Colleen Stockdale, Leonore Tiefer, and Yvette Trujillo (and many more).

This is the first book in which I have discussed aspects of my personal sexual life. For this, I am grateful to age, wisdom, and experience—and to those with whom I've been fortunate to fall in and out of like, love, lust, and crushes. The stories I've shared here are real, but identifying details have been omitted and sometimes changed in order to protect their privacy. They are good men I'm proud to have known and learned from, and with whom I enjoyed sharing parts of each other's lives.

I'm happy to have friends and family as sources of love and support. Ariane, Susie, Erica, Tom, Ben, Brooke, Brandon, Vanessa, Michael, Brian, Heather, Mike, David, Cathy, Mary, Susan, and Rick are among those whom I adore and whom I hope to always know (even if I don't see some of them nearly as much as I would like). My grandparents and parents provided a solid foundation for me that encouraged education and a sense of compassion and I will love them forever for that. I am grateful, too, to my sister Laura, my brother-in-law Tim, and my wonderful niece, who is a joy to be around and watch grow up into a bright, talented young woman. Finally, I want to express my most heartfelt joy to James (and to Jezebel), whom I can always count on for hugs, kisses, and cuddles. I appreciate his understanding when I interrupt dinner to email someone back with a response to a question about how to have an orgasm or last longer in bed. In my world, this happens more than I can say, and he's more patient and understanding than I could have hoped for.

Introduction

There is no such thing as a typical day of work for me—at least, not since I began working as a sex researcher, educator, and columnist at the Center for Sexual Health Promotion and the Kinsey Institute at Indiana University. Most days, I'm busy designing sex research studies (on topics such as women's orgasm, lubricant use, condom use, or sexual desire), analyzing data, writing research papers, grading students' exams or papers, writing sex columns, answering sex questions from journalists or television producers, or answering emails from students and colleagues. In my work as a sex columnist, I also read and answer emails from people who have questions about sex. Each month, I head into a recording studio on campus to tape a new batch of *Kinsey Confidential* audio podcasts. Occasionally, I'm sent products such as sex toys, lubricants, condoms, or arousal creams and am asked to provide input on their design, safety, or package instructions. With bookshelves lined with vulva puppets, vaginal dilators, sex toys, and books about sex, orgasm, and female ejaculation, it's not your normal office—and I wouldn't have it any other way.

Then there are days like a recent Friday, when a young woman made an appointment to ask for suggestions about how to overcome the pain she experienced every time she tried to have sex. The week before, a man called to ask about his erection difficulties. I think, too, of the married couple who were feeling distressed and, I think, a little sad about the wife's difficulty experiencing orgasm during intercourse. And it's a common occurrence for a student to stay after class to ask how to find the G Spot, whether it's normal to experience orgasms while doing sit-ups, or how to overcome premature ejaculation. Like I said, for me, there is no such thing as a typical day at work.

Women's and men's sex questions follow me everywhere and I welcome them. It was my grandmother who, several years before she died, best communicated to me how important it is to teach people about sex, bodies, and reproduction. At the time, I was twenty-three and had only recently started work at the Kinsey Institute. Knowing that she was quite religious and traditional, it took courage for me to tell her that I had started working at a place known for its pioneering research into human sexuality. Yet I didn't want to hide my job from her. When I finally took a deep breath and told her about my new job, she told me she thought it was important work and proceeded to tell me a story I had never heard before.

My grandmother told me that when she was pregnant with my mother, she didn't know how babies were delivered until she got to the hospital and was already going into labor. She had gone through her entire pregnancy assuming that her baby would eventually come out of her stomach because no one—not her girlfriends, sisters, or doctor (her mother had died when she was a teenager)—had told her otherwise. No one had mentioned anything about her baby being delivered through her vagina until the baby was ready to come out. Can you imagine the surprise, shock, and confusion that would cause? Because of that experience, my grandmother felt it was important that women and men be educated about their bodies and sexuality, and she was proud that I had accepted a research position at the Kinsey Institute, a place that had been central in opening up conversation and research about human sexuality. So here I am today, learning about sex and trying to make sure that rather than keep the information to myself, I share it with the world.

The Potential for Great Sex

I firmly believe that sex can be fantastic. Yet no one adequately prepares women or men to enjoy sex to its fullest. There's typically zero information about sexual pleasure included in most sex education programs, which means that people often learn about all the terrible things that can happen as part of sex (all the risks) but few of the very good things that can come from having sex. The lunacy of this tactic is that, most of the time, sex results in very good things, such as feelings of fun, pleasure, excitement, connection, intimacy, love, or even the chance to make a baby. The way we talk to each other about sex is broken and it's time we fix it. People want to know how to have fulfilling sex lives, not just how to keep bad things from happening. This book will answer that need.

As a result of my professional endeavors I have heard from probably a hundred thousand women and men about their sex lives. People have questions about every sex-related thing you can imagine (and many you've never dreamed of): questions about orgasm, pregnancy, painful sex, premature ejaculation, sex after baby, making sex more interesting, extending foreplay, low desire, birth control, fetishes, sex toys, the clitoris, desire discrepancy (when two members of a couple have different levels of desire), threesomes, erectile difficulties, monogamy, female ejaculation, oral sex, lasting longer, prostate stimulation, the G Spot, and much more.

Sometimes people write to me because they're excited about their sex lives, have a sexually generous partner, and are looking for tips to make sex even more exciting. Other times they write because they're feeling confused, "different," or alone in some way regarding sex. When I receive those kinds of letters and emails, I wish I could reply, "Sex doesn't have to be so hard." But sometimes it feels that way. It can be difficult not to take sexual problems to heart.

My feeling is that if we all knew more about sex, we could have happier, more pleasurable, more meaningful, and abundantly richer sex lives. They wouldn't be perfect, of course, but they would likely be easier and, at times, more fun.

As part of my work at Indiana University, I've had the pleasure of working on a number of interesting sex research studies. Of the dozens of studies I've conducted, the one that's received the greatest amount of popular press—and the one you have very likely read about—is called the National Survey of Sexual Health and Behavior (NSSHB). This study was only the second nationally representative study of the sexual behavior of Americans ever conducted. The first one took place in the early 1990s, before the Internet as we know it today even existed. It was nearly twenty years before researchers conducted another one (mostly due to a lack of funding for sex research in the US) and, thanks to support from Church & Dwight (the makers of Trojan condoms, vibrators, and other sexual health products), our Indiana University research team was able to conduct such a study. The NSSHB provided us with unique insights into Americans' sex lives: we got a glimpse into how many people engage in certain types of sex, the sexual difficulties people experience, and what makes sex more pleasurable or orgasmic for men and women. Here, in this book, I'll share many of the study's highlights with you.

Our research team has conducted a number of other important studies too, including those related to sexual desire, orgasm, and women's and men's use of sex toys, lubricant, and condoms. Between conducting research, writing about sex, teaching human sexuality classes, and attending conferences so I can learn from colleagues about their sex research studies, I spend a lot of time thinking about sex. Not only am I familiar with the many questions that women and men have, but I'm also intimately familiar with the answers (including trying to find answers to the sex mysteries that remain).

Sex in the Real World

Sex in the real world is complicated, and myths that oversimplify it can be harmful to people's lives, relationships, and marriages. You can love someone intensely but not click in the bedroom. You can be stunningly gorgeous and blessed with an equally hot partner yet still have disappointing, boring sex. There's also nothing unusual about you if you wonder about what it would be like to have sex with someone other than your relationship partner or spouse. And vibrators? More than half of women and about half of men use them. There's nothing strange about you if you use sex toys—or if you don't.

Whether you're struggling with sex or incredibly excited about sex and reading this because you're trying to make your sex life even better, there's something here for you. So how does sex improve? And what makes it easier? An important part of creating a satisfying, unforgettable sex life is learning about sex—something I cannot stress enough. If you commit to reading this book for ten or twenty minutes a day over the next few weeks or months, you will likely feel smarter and more confident about sex, and therefore more likely to have incredible sex.

Do Sex Experts Have Better Sex?

Because of what I do for work, I am often asked if studying and teaching about sex have made me better at *having* sex. Put another way, do sex experts have better sex? I can't speak for all sex experts, but I can speak for myself: studying sex has absolutely, 100 percent made me better at having not just any old sex, but wonderful sex.

None of us is born knowing how to have great sex. I knew next to nothing about sex for many years because my parents didn't know how to talk to my sister and me about it, my friends shared a lot of wrong information about it, and the teachers at my schools didn't teach us much about it either—that is, until I chose to return to school for a master's and PhD and learn everything I could about sex. However, I didn't just learn about sex in school; in addition to all the writing, teaching, and research activities I've already mentioned, I also learned about it by connecting with women who run in-home sex toy parties, listening to sexual health advocates, and talking with urologists, gynecologists, oncologists, dermatologists, and other doctors who focus on sexual medicine.

I now have a great deal of knowledge about sensitive body spots, creative sex positions, sexual health, and sexual pleasure—and I don't take any of this for granted. I believe it is my duty (and my privilege) to share this knowledge with those who want to better their own sex lives.

One of the most important lessons I've learned is this: research shows that most people will face sexual difficulties sooner or later, even small ones like experiencing genital burning from a vagina-unfriendly lubricant or finding enough time or energy for sex. Thanks to kids, pets, work, families, stress, and laundry lists of things to do, life sometimes gets in the way. The difference is that, as someone who knows about sex, when problems happen to me I have a sense of how to respond: what to do and what *not* to do. I won't freak out, get mad, or blame myself or my partner for the numerous little sexual problems that can feel big and scary to those who haven't yet learned much about sex. Instead, I know where to turn and what to try, and I have a better sex life for it. It's not a perfect sex life, but it's one I enjoy and am thankful for.

What I'm sharing here in this book can do the same for you. When you reach beyond the empty sex promises and myths we've all been sold, you have the chance to start your own at-home sex revolution. More satisfying sex can be yours if you spend a little bit of time learning about it and putting your new knowledge and skills into (very fun) practice.

The *Sex Made Easy* approach is basically this: if you learn about sex, you're likely to feel more excited and confident being naked, having fun with your partner, tackling sex challenges together, taking care of your sexual health, and maybe even enjoying a few more orgasms than usual.

I don't have all the answers, but I have enough answers and many creative, sex-positive ideas that add up to a great sex life. This book is about having knowledge, skills, and confidence to have a sex life that feels good and that doesn't bring panic, blame, or shame into the bedroom. It's about moving toward sex that helps you enjoy what you have, not worry about what's missing, fix what can be fixed, and talk comfortably with your partner about everything that's going on. It's also about not feeling so isolated, alone, or "abnormal" for having sex problems in the first place (we all have them from time to time).

What to Expect

In the pages that follow, you will find plenty of information about bodies and sex as well as a hundred sex questions and concerns I've heard from women and men just like you. Some of these are very common questions (for example, about having an orgasm or lasting longer) whereas others are less common (for example, questions about coregasms or sex-related headaches). I've even included some of the less common questions because it can be difficult to find trustworthy information about these issues and I believe that people who have these concerns deserve to have access to information that may help them. Also, some of them are just plain curious and interesting.

I'm also doing something in this book that I have never done before: I'm sharing stories from my own trials and errors on the road to good sex. I thought for a long time about whether or not I wanted to go there, but I think it's important that more of us start being honest about our sex lives rather than pretend that everything is always perfect. Hopefully, when we're honest about the complexities of love and sex, we can all feel more normal and relaxed and know we're not alone with our problems.

Like I said, nearly everyone has (or will have) sex problems and that includes sex experts like me. Knowing about sex doesn't inoculate a person from having issues, but it does help prepare one to address them in order to create a happier sex life. By sharing these problems and solutions, I hope to arm you with enough knowledge to tackle your own sex issues and enough hope to see that even difficult sex problems can often be managed successfully.

Finally, although not all sex problems are "easy" to fix—and I certainly don't mean to suggest that with the title of this book—almost any sex problem can be made easier to deal with if one has knowledge about the issue it involves, or simply a sense that others have been down this road too and sex (or one's relationship) will likely get better. It can also be helpful to distinguish between what you can handle on your own versus what you need outside help with: it's the difference between knowing if your baby's fever can be treated at home or if she requires a visit to the pediatrician, or between knowing if you can fix your leaky faucet yourself or need to call a plumber. After reading *Sex Made Easy*, I expect that you will have a better sense of what, in the bedroom, you can fix on your own versus when you should call a doctor or therapist. I also expect that you'll be eager to go out and have a whole lot of fun in and out of bed. Ready?

Let's begin.

CHAPTER 1

Vulvalicious: Your Down-There Guide to Better Sex

When comedian Chelsea Handler's book *Chelsea Chelsea Bang Bang* was first published, I was excited to read her newest stories. That excitement, however, soon turned to appreciation mixed with disappointment when I opened her book to "The Feeling," a story about how Chelsea learned to masturbate at a sleepover party with her childhood girlfriends.[1]

My appreciation stemmed from the fact that Chelsea had courageously written about a sensitive topic (female sexuality remains taboo to talk about at any age, but people particularly tiptoe around it when discussing children even though young girls and boys commonly explore their own bodies.[2]) My disappointment, however, stemmed from how Chelsea wrote about looking at her vulva, which she calls her "coslopus" (one of the more inventive and vague terms for "vulva" that I've so far encountered). She wrote about looking at her vulva and initially feeling "disgust," compounded with the "horrific news" that women eventually develop pubic hair. I kept hoping she'd write about transforming her horror/disgust/disdain into some adolescent or adult vulva appreciation or even adoration—kind of like how, in *Beauty and the Beast*, Belle comes to love the Beast. I hoped that she'd write about coming to appreciate her vulva not only for the pleasurable aspects of masturbation (which she describes enormous appreciation of) but for the way the vulva looks or feels, even when it's just sitting there being a plain old vulva. Yet I can't and don't blame Chelsea. Many people of both sexes aren't too thrilled with what's between their legs. Granted, I happen to think vulvas, penises, and scrotums are awesome, but I didn't always feel that way. I, too, was once perplexed about my parts, not to mention boys' parts.

A Genital Education

Having no brothers, the first time I saw a penis (that I can recall, anyway) wasn't until kindergarten. We had assigned seats in our classroom and I sat with the same group of friends every day. One morning while coloring worksheets, the kids at my table began looking underneath the table and giggling. Someone told me to look, so I did. Peeking underneath the table, I saw that a boy at my table had pulled aside the crotch of his shorts and his underwear.

Why is he holding a baby bottle nipple in between his legs? I wondered, not realizing that boys' parts were different from girls' parts and that what he was holding wasn't a baby bottle nipple at all but his five-year-old penis.

I kept staring, confused at the curious placement of this baby bottle, when one of the girls at my table said, through her giggles, that it was his penis (though she probably called it something like "wee wee" or "wiener"). As much as I adore penises now, at the time there was nothing in me that clamored for more penis sightings or thought that this penis thing was great. It looked weird to me—and definitely more like a baby bottle nipple than a body part.

Early experiences looking at my own genitals were surprising, though I don't ever remember thinking of them as "weird" (curious and puzzling, yes, but not in a bad way). As a child, I remember looking at and touching my genitals out of curiosity and to "de-fuzz" them. Specifically, I recall touching my clitoris, even though at the time I definitely didn't know its name or what it was for. All I remember is that, for some reason, I was looking at it while sitting on the family room sofa and I noticed that there were cotton fuzzies (from my underwear) stuck in the folds of my clitoris and I was trying to get them out. I recall that this funny, wrinkly looking body part was sensitive to touch, and I thus had to de-fuzz it very carefully—almost as carefully as the time I tried to remove the pink sticky bubble gum I'd accidentally dropped from my mouth onto my black Persian cat's furry head (poor thing).

When my mom walked in on my careful and conscientious de-fuzzing, I think she asked what I was doing or told me not to touch down there or that it was dirty to touch myself there or something along those lines. Her reaction wasn't mean; I think she was simply surprised to walk in and find me de-fuzzing my clitoris (and who can blame her? I was doing this on the family room sofa!). Now, in my work as a sex educator, I regularly hear similar stories from parents of young children: parents whose daughters absentmindedly touch their genitals while reading the Sunday comics, or who rub against their security blanket because, they say, it makes them feel "happy." These parents wonder how to respond to their kids and ask if they should ignore these instances or use them as "teachable moments" to teach their daughters and sons about their bodies. (In case you find yourself in a similar situation as a parent, common advice is to respond by saying something like "That's okay to do, but you should do it somewhere private, such as in your bedroom or in the bathroom." This acknowledges the behavior, yet doesn't suggest that self-touching is dirty or shameful, only that it is better done in private.)

In my case, it would be many years before I learned more about women's and men's genitals, including how to love and appreciate these body parts for what they are and what they have the potential to do and feel. Many years after the childhood de-fuzzing incident, when I was a teenager, I checked my vulva out simply because I was curious about it and my vagina (though I didn't know what a vulva was and how it was different from my vagina until my early twenties). By my late teens, I had heard a great deal about sex and I wondered how it was all supposed to happen, this penis-in-the-vagina business. Looking in a mirror, I noticed how small my vaginal opening looked and wondered how a penis was ever supposed to fit inside there one day. I had no immediate plans for intercourse; I was simply curious.

Given my own personal experiences and my later experiences working as a sex educator, hearing from so many young and adult women who have questions about their bodies, I believe that we (educators, parents, and teachers) should do a better job of giving young women helpful information about their bodies. If they are educated, they won't have to wonder about or be afraid of how their vagina will manage childbirth (remember the story about my grandmother from the introduction?), tampon use, or vaginal intercourse. The ways vaginas can lubricate and expand seems like good information to share with young women and men. As a fourth grader, I recall being fascinated to learn how the lungs, heart, kidneys, pancreas, liver, and other body parts work; that doesn't mean I was determined to put what I learned to the test. Perhaps teaching young women and men how vulvas, vaginas, penises, and scrotums work would be of value too. Then maybe fewer of us would be fearful, ashamed, or, as Chelsea Handler put it, *disgusted* when we check out our genitals. Maybe we would even celebrate them.

The Great Wall of Vagina

In 2011, UK sculptor Jamie McCartney unveiled plaster casts of the vulvas of four hundred women in an effort to provide a glimpse into how wonderfully diverse we women are between our legs. As he says on his website, "It's not vulgar, it's vulva!" He also writes, "For many women their genital appearance is a source of anxiety and I was in a unique position to do something about that." Good for him. Check it out at http://www.greatwallofvagina.co.uk.

KNOW YOUR PARTS: A GUIDED TOUR

Whether you call your vulva "down there," "pussy," or—like Chelsea Handler—your "coslopus" (a name I can never remember; it sounds too much like the *Sesame Street* character Snuffleupagus), I hope you call it something. I also hope you check it out from time to time.

If you haven't seen your vulva very often, or if you've seen it but aren't sure you know all the part names, let's take a quick tour. And in case the word "vulva" is new to you, it refers to a woman's external genitals, the parts a woman can see when she's naked and her legs are apart, like what the doctor sees during a GYN (gynecology) exam. Try using it in a sentence like this:

- "I love my vulva."
- "My boyfriend loves licking my vulva."

- "The clitoris is my favorite part of my girlfriend's vulva."
- "The masturbation sleeve I bought my husband looks like a vulva."
- "*The Vagina Monologues* isn't just filled with vagina stories—there are plenty of vulva stories in there too."
- "Every month, I examine my vulva to make sure things are healthy and happy down there."

Now back to our guided tour. Although you can follow along with our diagram, you can also follow along with your own vulva if you have one (or if your ready-and-willing partner has one). Got a vulva? Good. That plus a well-lit space and a mirror will make it easier to give yourself a tour.

Starting at the top is the mons pubis, which might have a triangular tuft of hair—or at least it usually has hair, though some women shave or wax off their pubic hair. The mons can be seen when you're standing around naked. To see the rest of the vulva, slightly open your legs. Get a mirror and make sure you have decent light. There at the top is the clitoral hood. Between the hood and the glans clitoris (what most people just call "the clitoris" even though there's a lot more to the clitoris that's inside the body; the clitoris has two branches that extend several inches inside the

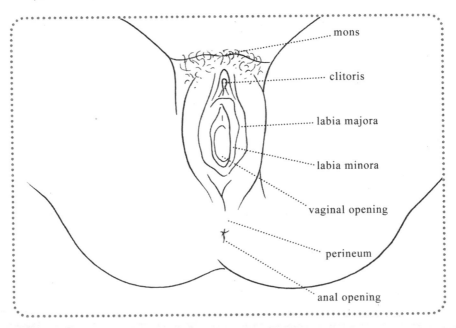

body and that may be stimulated during vaginal intercourse) is the part where **smegma** and other things, like fuzzies from cotton underwear, sometimes get stuck. Smegma is made by women's and men's bodies and often hides out in the folds of the genitals. It's basically a collection of skin cells and oils produced by the body and may look white or grayish. It's a totally normal bodily production and nothing to be ashamed of. Think of it as the vagina's version of eye crusties or ear wax; we all make it.

Framing the **vaginal opening** (which may look very small even if you've had vaginal intercourse or delivered a baby) are two sets of labia, also called vaginal lips. The **labia majora,** also called the **outer lips,** usually have hair on the outer side and are hairless on the inside. They may be larger or smaller than the **labia minora** (also called the **inner labia**), which are hairless. Some women have such tiny inner labia that they can barely even see them. Other women have inner labia that, when they stand up, are long enough to hang below the outer labia. Every woman is different and no labia setup is better or worse. The inner labia often have several shades of color to them: shades of pink, red, lavender, brown, gray, or black. Like many flower petals (for example, orchid petals), it's common for the labia to be framed with darker edges, giving them a pretty, textured appearance. Your labia are your labia: they don't get bigger or smaller no matter how much sex or masturbation you engage in. They may, however, grow slightly larger during sexual arousal as blood flow increases to them. Woman's inner labia may also grow larger during pregnancy, thanks to hormonal changes and increases in blood flow. And with advanced age, they may grow smaller or more wrinkly, like other body parts. Other than these normal developmental changes, labia are what they are and they're a little different for each one of us.

Below the vaginal area is the **perineum,** which is the area in between the bottom of the vaginal entrance and the anal opening. The perineum feels sensitive for some women. For some, this sensitivity may be uncomfortable, particularly if they have had scar tissue develop in the perineal area because there has been tearing from childbirth or an episiotomy (a surgical procedure that involves cutting the perineum during birth).

LUMPS, BUMPS, DISCHARGE, AND TEARING

As wonderful as the vulva has the potential to be, it can also be quite sensitive. A woman's estrogen supply helps keep the vulva and vagina strong. When a woman has lower levels of estrogen due to menopause, breastfeeding, or various health conditions, her vulva and vagina may be more prone to tearing. Certain genital skin conditions can also make a woman's vulva more prone to tearing, including tearing during sex. Women who tear frequently during sex would be wise to mention this to their health care provider, who can investigate whether this is a result of lack of estrogen or some other health issue.

In addition to small cuts and tears, women also sometimes notice lumps and bumps on their genitals—as do many men. In most cases, these lumps and bumps aren't anything to worry about. Some are moles, just like the moles that may be found on other body parts. Small bumps can also result from mild razor burn or irritated hair follicles, and often heal quickly on their own. In some cases, however, a bump may be a genital wart, caused by strains of the human papillomavirus (HPV). In very rare cases, a bump on the vulva may be a sign of vulvar cancer. By performing monthly vulvar self-examination (VSE, which basically entails checking out each of your vulva parts at least once each month), you can increase your chances of catching tricky things early.[3] As with any other body part, if you let your health care provider know about any lumps, bumps, itchy spots, or changes in skin color that you find on your vulva (such as white or dark patches of skin), you'll be in a better position to get help early.

Labia "Puff" Procedures

As far as plastic surgery is concerned, it seems no body part is left without options. In 2011 I was surprised to learn of a genital procedure being touted as the "labia puff" procedure. This involves using injections to make the labia majora (the outer labia) appear slightly larger or perhaps less wrinkled (in the sense that the injected fillers are intended to fill in any sagging labia tissue). While some surgeons insist they are simply offering women options for enhancing their self-image, others challenge the idea of making so many tweaks to women's already beautiful bodies. Some groups, such as the New View Campaign, aim to raise awareness of what is described on its website as "the unregulated and unmonitored genital cosmetic surgery industry." The New View Campaign has staged protests of female genital cosmetic surgery; it has also held conferences and art exhibits that aim to celebrate the diversity of women's genitals. Learn more at http://www.newviewcampaign.org/fgcs.asp.

A HAIRY SITUATION

No matter what you read in magazines or hear from your friends, let me be clear: there is no one dominant "everybody's doing it" pubic hairstyle. How do I know this? Because my research team at Indiana University was one of the first groups to do a study on the topic and it involved asking more than twenty-four hundred women in the US about their pubic hairstyles.[4]

We found that women do any number of things to their pubic hair, including rock these styles:

• **Totally natural.** Also called a "full bush," "retro bush," or "hipster bush," this style involves nothing other than working with what Mother Nature gave you. For some women, this is a small amount of hair, mostly on the pubic mound. For others, there may be a large amount of hair extending above the pubic mound and onto the upper thighs.

• **Trimmed.** Some women find that smaller scissors help them to get in close to carefully trim their pubic hair. I know of one woman who was into crafting and discovered that her smallest pair of scissors (the kind commonly used in kindergarten classes) was the easiest to use when trimming her pubes.

• **Fashioned.** Women fashion their pubic hair into all sorts of different designs (for example, their or their partner's first initial, a heart, star, or V for vulva or vagina), with the landing strip—roughly a one-inch-thick vertical strip of hair—being one of the more common ones. This is usually done by shaving the hair around the shape that's meant to be left on, though some salons specialize in waxing women's pubic hair into preferred designs. In our 2010 study, removing only some pubic hair (as opposed to all of it) was the most common thing women did to their pubic hair, with about 29 percent of women ages eighteen to twenty-four, 39 percent of women ages twenty-five to twenty-nine, and 50 percent of women in their thirties and forties saying they had shaved or waxed some of their hair in the previous month but they hadn't gone bare.

• **Bare.** Taking it all off can be done through shaving or waxing. Some women enjoy the smooth feel of their hairless vulva. Others think that's fine and dandy, but the stubbly process of growing it back in isn't for them. And while some women say that having a bare vulva makes them feel too much like a prepubescent child, others feel sexy and grown-up when bare. In our study, women who had mostly gone bare in the past month were more likely to be young (college aged) or bisexual-identified, or to have recently engaged in cunnilingus.

There's a lot of hype about how women wear their down-there hair. Some magazines make it sound like every woman in America is bare, and that's just not the case. In our study we found that only 20.6 percent of women ages eighteen to twenty-four were typically bare down there. This number dropped significantly to only about 12.4 percent of women ages twenty-five to twenty-nine, 8.6 percent of women in their thirties, 6.5 percent of women in their forties, and 2 percent of women age fifty or older. That's not to say that the rest of the women didn't sometimes remove all of their hair, or that they never had, but it's safe to say that it was more common for a woman to keep at least some of her pubic hair than to get rid of it.

PUBIC HAIR AND PLEASURE

In 2008, a team of researchers set out to understand the curious nature of women's hair removal.[5] They asked 235 female undergraduate students in Australia a number of questions about their removal of underarm, leg, and pubic hair, including complete removal of pubic hair. Women indicated that some of the most important reasons why they removed their underarm and leg hair were these: all of their friends do it; it's expected of them; people "would look at (them) funny" if they didn't; and they thought that men preferred women without body hair. These women also strongly indicated that they removed their leg and underarm hair because it made them feel sexy, feminine, cleaner, confident, and good about themselves—reasons that were also largely given for removing some or all of their pubic hair. Women who removed some or all of their pubic hair also generally said that they felt it made their sexual experiences better.

When we set out to conduct our pubic hair study, we were curious about the issue of sex: namely, would there be differences in sexual function for women based on what they did with their pubic hair? We found that even after we statistically controlled for age, sexual relationship status, and sexual orientation, women who removed all of their pubic hair—even just once—in the preceding month scored higher on several measures of sexual function. Put another way, women who went bare tended to report higher desire, higher arousal, less pain during sex, greater sexual satisfaction, and greater vaginal lubrication during sex. We found no differences in regard to orgasm.

This doesn't mean that ditching your pubic hair will change your sex life. Then again, maybe there is something about the process of going bare that tunes women in to their bodies more, or that arouses them during the process (or later, when their genitals are more noticeable to them or their partner). Anecdotally, women describe diverse feelings about their pubic hair. Some have told me that they like having pubic hair, especially full "tufts" of pubic hair, because it helps to cushion intercourse and make it feel more comfortable. Some women prefer to trim or wax, rather than shave, given how uncomfortable stubble can feel as hair grows back in.

The take-home message when it comes to pubic hair is that you should do what you like, what makes you feel comfortable, and maybe what makes you feel sexy—if feeling sexy is important to you. The nice thing about pubic hairstyles is that you can change them at any time. If you go bare and dislike it, you can grow it back. If you trim your pubic hair too short, give it a few days and it will grow longer again. And if you're tired of too-long hairs, then trim, wax, or shave. It's your hair, so do what you like and don't let anyone tell you otherwise.

THE VAGINA

Whole entire books have been written about the vagina and if you have tons of questions about this wonderful body part, I suggest you check out my earlier book, *Read My Lips: A Complete Guide to the Vagina and Vulva (2011)* or *The V Book: A Doctor's Guide to Complete Vulvovaginal Health* (2002) by Elizabeth Stewart and Paula Spencer. Here we will stick to some of the most basic things you need to know about your vagina as it relates to better sex.

First, the vagina is the inside part, also known as the birth canal. Second, the vagina is only about three or four inches long, though it can get longer and wider when a woman becomes sexually aroused (a process called vaginal tenting). Third, it needs attention! At least once each year, or as often as your health care provider recommends, bring your vagina (and the rest of you) in for an annual gynecological exam. Fourth, the vagina has simple tastes; it neither needs nor wants to be covered with douches, deodorants, baby powder, or fragranced bath soap. Fifth, the vagina is surrounded by pelvic floor muscles that help to support your genitals and other internal organs. These same muscles can help to enhance sensation during sex. Many women do **Kegel exercises** (pronounced "kay-gull") to

- Help strengthen the pelvic floor muscles
- Support the internal organs
- Reduce the risk of incontinence that comes with childbearing and older age, and
- Maintain vaginal sensation during sex

Here's how you do Kegel exercises. First, identify your pelvic floor muscles by squeezing as if you're trying to stop yourself from peeing midstream. Or insert one finger into your vagina and squeeze it. Feel that? Good. Now that you've found your pelvic floor muscles, it's time to put them to work. Squeeze them for ten seconds, then release the squeeze and let them relax for ten seconds. Repeat this over and over again for five or ten minutes at least once per day. You might also want to ask your health care provider if he or she has any favorite Kegel exercise "routines"; providers vary, and some recommend holding them for longer, squeezing and releasing more quickly and rhythmically, or doing them more than once a day.

Just as health care providers vary, so do women: if you are a woman who experiences vaginal or vulvar pain, check in with your health care provider or a physical therapist who specializes in genital pain disorders before starting a Kegel exercise routine, as some experts believe that some genital pain conditions may be caused or made worse by pelvic floor muscles that are already too tight.

Another important aspect (the sixth thing on our list) pertains to **vaginal lubrication.** As women become sexually aroused, blood flows to their genitals. This causes fluids to pass through their blood vessels and through the walls of the vagina to create vaginal lubrication. A woman's estrogen levels also influence her vaginal lubrication,[6] and women with higher estrogen levels tend to find that they lubricate more quickly and more easily than women with lower estrogen levels, such as those who are menopausal or breastfeeding.

THE G SPOT

Everyone, it seems, wants to know about the G Spot. Every semester that I teach human sexuality, men and women alike want to know how to find the G Spot and whether it really exists. Readers of my sex columns write to ask how to know whether or not they have a G Spot in the first place or how to stimulate their partner's G Spot. Here's what you need to know.

The G Spot got its name in the 1980s and pays homage to Dr. Ernst

Grafenberg who, back in the 1950s, described an area along the front vaginal wall that—when stimulated—is erotically sensitive for some but not all women. The G Spot is often described as being located about two inches inside the vagina on the front vaginal wall. Women can try to locate it themselves although sometimes, given the angle of stimulating one's own vagina, it can be easier to have one's partner attempt G Spot exploration using one's fingers or penis or a sex toy. Although sex toy companies make G Spot vibrators and dildos that are curved for easier stimulation of the front wall, one does not need a G Spot vibrator or dildo for G Spot play. Fingers, a penis, or a non-curved sex toy work just as well (as long as the vibrator or dildo is made for vaginal insertion).

The G Spot remains controversial even among sex researchers. There hasn't been much scientific research conducted on the G Spot and what has been done has shed only a little bit of light on the topic. One researcher in a 2001 article published in the *American Journal of Obstetrics & Gynecology* went as far as to describe the G Spot as "a modern gynecologic myth"[7] given that the existing research at the time was mostly based on small samples of women and in some cases was difficult to interpret. The issue was further muddled when, in 2008, Italian researchers published an article in the *Journal of Sexual Medicine* claiming that ultrasonography could be used to identify the G Spot in women.[8] They based this on data from a study that involved only twenty women. The researchers suggested that the space between the urethra and vagina was thicker among the nine women in their study who reported experiencing vaginal orgasm compared to the eleven-women who reported not having vaginal orgasms and; on this basis, they felt that they had "found" the G Spot. This study made headlines in magazines and on blogs and yet, in the opinion of a number of scientists (myself included), it was flawed—not only because it involved so few women but because it is difficult to determine who has "vaginal orgasms" and who does not. The researchers had simply asked women "Have you ever experienced a vaginal orgasm?" Based on this question alone, I am not certain that they would have successfully been able to separate women into groups of who had and who had not had a vaginal orgasm.

The whole idea of a "vaginal orgasm" is contested territory. Because the clitoris has branches that extend backward into the body, some researchers believe that vaginal stimulation likely stimulates the clitoris too. There is also evidence that the vagus nerve, which carries sensory information from the cervix, is one pathway to orgasm. Because one cannot easily stimulate the cervix without stimulating the vagina too, it's likely that multiple parts of a woman's body are stimulated during vaginal intercourse, fingering, or sex toy play. Can we really put women's orgasms into neat little boxes of vaginal orgasms, clitoral orgasms, G Spot orgasms, and so on? Probably not.

Two years after the Italian study was published, another study was published also in the *Journal of Sexual Medicine* that claimed the there was no evidence for the G Spot.[9] How did they come to this conclusion? They asked women in their study, "Do you believe you have a so-called G Spot …?" They didn't examine the women. They didn't ask detailed follow-up questions about their sexual experiences, orgasms, or experiences with G Spot stimulation. Nor did they acknowledge in the article that the use of the phrase "so-called" may have biased or influenced their participants. I was at a scientific meeting when one of the researchers presented the study and was met with a great deal of criticism from other scientists who questioned whether the study was able to answer the question of whether or not the G Spot existed (most scientists who spoke out did not feel the study could adequately address the issue).

Perhaps you can see the challenge the G Spot presents, even among scientific circles. One day, scientists say, "Eureka, we've found it!" and the next, another team of scientists says "Not so fast—we've just proven it doesn't exist!" and the cycle continues. Of course, this is both the blessing and the curse of science. Most important discoveries are not instant "Eureka!" moments. In science, it often takes a number of studies—and often significant disagreement and then fine-tuning of subsequent studies—to produce greater knowledge.

As such, here is how I like to think of the G Spot: Based on the scientific evidence that we do have, I believe that many, but not all, women have an area on the front wall of the vagina that, when stimulated, feels good to them. All women who have vaginas have this area, but not all women enjoy being stimulated there (this is true of any body part: women have a clitoris and breasts too, but not all women find clitoral stimulation or breast stimulation to be pleasurable or orgasmic). The G Spot can be stimulated through intercourse positions (missionary with one's hips tilted upward is a popular position for G Spot stimulation, as is woman on top). It can also be explored through finger play (two fingers using gentle but firm stimulation is often recommended) or through sex toy play (again, a G Spot–specific toy is not necessary). As for whether "G Spot orgasms" (orgasms that result from stimulation of the G Spot) feel different from other orgasms, it seems to depend on the woman. Some women prefer G Spot stimulation over other types of stimulation, such as clitoral stimulation. Others prefer clitoral stimulation over G Spot stimulation. My advice is to explore your body and find what feels good to you.

Love Hurts, but Should Sex?

The answer, of course, is no; sex should not hurt. However, sex is often painful for women. In the National Survey of Sexual Health and Behavior that my research team conducted, we found that about 30 percent of women experienced some degree of pain the most recent time they had sex, compared to about 5 percent of men.[10] That's a huge difference! If you're raising a teenaged or young adult daughter, make sure she knows that although sex sometimes hurts the first time or two, it shouldn't keep hurting. If it does, she should see her health care provider. And if sex hurts for you, check in with your health care provider. Also connect with the National Vulvodynia Association (www.nva.org) for additional resources and, if needed, doctor referrals.

— Making It Easy —

1. What to do if . . . one labium is bigger than the other

In most women, one labium (the singular term for labia; a woman's vaginal lip) is bigger than the other. This is very common and nothing to feel embarrassed about. Not only is one labium often a different size and shape from its pair (even the coloration can vary) but women's labia can look more or less symmetrical depending on how a woman sits or how she or her partner hold her labia. Think of how your face looks in a photograph depending on the angle the picture is taken from. The vulva is similar in this regard. So if you're not thrilled by how your labia stack up, remember that they probably look completely different from another angle. If you don't believe me, grab a mirror and see for yourself.

Most of the time, differently shaped labia are just that—differently shaped. They're not better or worse than labia of the same size. With few exceptions, labia size typically doesn't affect how a woman pees, has babies, or enjoys sex. In very rare cases, one or both labia may be large enough to cause pain or discomfort for a woman when she has sex, rides a bike, takes long walks, wears certain clothing, or performs other daily activities. In such cases, health care providers sometimes recommend a procedure called a labiaplasty, which is a resizing and reshaping of one or both labia.

Labiaplasty has become a controversial procedure as some women, health care providers, and women's health advocates worry that in recent years the procedure has been unnecessarily, and sometimes unethically, marketed toward women. Because any surgery carries risks, if you are considering labiaplasty, I would recommend checking in with a health care provider who specializes in vaginal and vulvar health issues and who has the best interests of you and your body in mind. You can find such a provider through the International Society for the Study of Vulvovaginal Disease (www.issvd.org). This isn't to say that all labiaplasty is bad; some women feel better about their bodies and are more easily able to participate in sex (or exercise) after labiaplasty. Rather, I simply encourage you to seek out quality information before having surgery done on any body part, including the vulva.

You might also find it of interest to know about a study published in 2011 in the *Journal of Sexual Medicine:* in a recent survey of medical doctors, male doctors and plastic surgeons were significantly more likely to describe normal labia as "unnatural" and say they would recommend labiaplasty for women with normal-looking labia than were female doctors, gynecologists, and general practitioners.[11] In other words, if you have questions about your labia, you might be better off asking a female gynecologist or a general practitioner—or at least including one such doctor as a second or third opinion—before going under the knife. It also sounds like medical schools might want to do a better job of educating future doctors about the wide range of normal, beautiful, healthy vulvas and their labia. You might find it helpful to ask yourself why (or if) it matters that one labium is longer or bigger than the other: our bodies aren't symmetrical in any other place; why would this place be symmetrical? Are there things about your life that you think might be different if your labia were the same size? How might that work? And what if that's not the case?

2. What to do if . . . you get ingrown pubic hairs but want to keep removing your pubic hair

Many women are susceptible to razor bumps or ingrown hairs on their body, including on their pubic area. Some women who are tired of dealing with repeated ingrown hairs choose to stop removing their pubic hair and instead opt for trimming it. Others choose laser hair reduction, as it is more permanent, though there's no guarantee of complete removal. In other words, if your goal is to go completely bare down there, repeated laser hair reduction may be able to help you permanently remove many of your pubic hairs, but you may never be completely pubic hair–free. An advantage of laser treatment, however, is that it destroys the hair follicle; this can lead to fewer bumps and ingrown hairs. If you prefer to keep shaving, you may be able to lower the risk of razor bumps and ingrown hairs by taking a hot shower or bath before shaving to soften your pubic hairs and help open the pores in your skin. Try shaving in the same direction of hair growth too, which is the opposite of how many women shave their legs.

Razor bumps frustrate some people when it comes to sex because the bumps may make them feel less sexy. Dimming the light or using candlelight to illuminate the bedroom can minimize the appearance of razor bumps and ingrowns. Or, you can remind yourself that we're all human, we all have skin issues from time to time, and your partner is lucky to be with you just as you are with them, razor bumps or not. That said, if your bumps truly are from shaving or ingrown hairs, you may want to bring the issue up and reassure your partner about what caused them, lest they wonder whether you have a sexually transmitted infection (STI) or some other infection. (And if you do have an STI, I hope you will find a way to share this with your partner, as it's the kind thing to do.)

3. What to do if . . . sex hurts at first (but not when you keep going)

If sex hurts for you, mention this to a health care provider. A gynecologist, in particular, is a good place to start, as he or she can examine your vagina, cervix, and vulva (the outside parts) to look for an identifiable reason. Often if sex hurts only when penetration begins but then gets better, a lack of lubrication and time spent in foreplay is to blame. It can take several minutes after a woman feels sexually aroused—even as long as ten to twenty minutes—for her to produce enough vaginal lubrication for comfortable penetration. It can also take this long for a woman's body to become sufficiently aroused so that her vagina grows longer and wider (vaginal tenting), thus making more room inside for comfortable penetration with a partner's fingers, a sex toy, or a partner's penis.

One strategy, then, is to spend longer in foreplay doing whatever it is that makes you feel tingly, sexy, and excited before starting vaginal penetration or intercourse. A sex therapist I know told me that she would advise women to wait to begin intercourse until the vagina felt like it was practically throbbing for sex. That level of sexual excitement is often a good indication that a woman is sufficiently aroused and her vaginal lubrication is in good supply.

If you'd rather not wait to start sex for whatever reason (quickies can be fun too), you might try applying a dab of water-based lubricant to your vaginal entrance as well as to the fingers, penis, or sex toy that's about to enter you. That might make for more comfortable sex. If extra foreplay and added lubricant don't ease your pain, circle back with your doctor and ask what else might be causing it. If your doctor can't figure it out, get a second opinion from a doctor who specializes in vaginal and vulvar health.

4. What to do if . . . sex hurts the entire time

As I've said before, any time sex hurts, you should mention this to a health care provider, such as a gynecologist. If your gynecologist isn't able to determine what's at the bottom of your pain, consider getting a second opinion from a vulvovaginal specialist or a dermatologist. That's right—a dermatologist, a doctor who specializes in skin health and disease. Dermatologists and gynecologists have different specialized kinds of training and one type of doctor sometimes picks up on certain health conditions that the other type misses. In the case of genital pain, some cases of painful sex are caused by skin disorders that affect women's genitals. Some skin disorders can cause women's genital skin to become very thin and easy to tear during sex. A dermatologist can help rule out skin conditions that might be contributing to genital pain.

As I mentioned before, spending more time in foreplay and adding water-based lubricant may be helpful. And if you're approaching menopause, are postmenopausal, if you've had your ovaries removed (perhaps as part of a hysterectomy or for other reasons), or if you've undergone cancer treatments that have affected how your ovaries function, then you might benefit from using a vaginal moisturizer; ask your health care provider if this is a good choice for you. Some vaginal moisturizers contain estrogens but not all do. Vaginal moisturizers are different from lubricants in that they help the vagina maintain a level of wetness for days on end and aren't just used during sex. Vaginal moisturizers are typically used two or three times a week and may be inserted into the vagina at night before bed, where they are left to do their work while you sleep. If you are recently sexually active after a long absence of sex, or after having had some type of vaginal surgery, ask your health care provider whether vaginal dilator therapy is right for you.

Vaginal Dilators

Vaginal dilators can be thought of as "medical dildos" in the sense that they look like dildos (not the kind that are penis-shaped though) but they tend to be recommended by health care providers and therapists for therapeutic use. Vaginal dilators are typically sold in sets of five or six, with the smallest being about the size of one's little finger and the largest being larger than the average-sized penis. Dilators are often recommended for use by women experiencing vaginal pain or difficulty with penetration, for any number of health reasons. Doctors and therapists who recommend that their patients use dilators tend to suggest starting with the smallest size first and slowly (over a period of weeks or months) working one's way up to larger sizes.

I recommend dilators that are somewhat soft and flexible, with some "give" to them for easier insert. I also recommend choosing dilators that are made of materials that are easy to clean and preferably smooth along the sides, without noticeable seams, for comfortable insertion. I helped design, and do not profit from, a set of dilators that are available from http://pureromance.com. This particular set has the important features I just described and can make dilator use more comfortable and hygienic. However, as many health care providers and therapists will tell you, one can also use differently sized candlesticks (with a condom covering them) or one's own fingers, beginning with the smallest finger. Using water-based lubricant with vaginal dilators (or dildos, candlesticks, or your own fingers) can make penetration easier and more comfortable. Keep in mind, too, that one needn't do "in and out" thrusting motions with them. Many women insert the lubricated dilator an inch or two (or more) inside their vagina and let it sit there while they read a book, check email, or watch television. The idea is to teach one's vagina to comfortably accept penetration over time.

5. What to do if . . . you feel constantly aroused, even after masturbating, having sex, or having orgasms

Although it's uncommon, some women experience sexual arousal for hours, days, or months without relief, even after masturbating or having sex with one or more orgasms. Some women enjoy this experience of ongoing sexual arousal; others do not. They may find it uncomfortable or distracting, especially if it's not part of a bigger experience of feeling sexually aroused or desirous.

First described in 2001, this was initially called Persistent Sexual Arousal Syndrome and was more recently renamed Persistent Genital Arousal Disorder (PGAD), as women with PGAD are more likely to say that their genitals are feeling "aroused" (rather than that they feel sexually aroused themselves).[12] It's unclear what causes PGAD. Some women report that their symptoms started either while taking certain antidepressants or after they stopped taking antidepressants. One study reported on a woman who started experiencing PGAD about a month after she started on a diet that was very, very high in soy (her genital arousal was so unrelenting that she would masturbate upwards of fifteen times in a day to try to relieve the tension).[13] Other research suggests that women with PGAD are more likely to be anxious or depressed and to monitor their physical sensations (how their body feels), suggesting that perhaps these psychological characteristics are linked to PGAD.[14] This doesn't mean that PGAD is "all in your head"; rather, women who pay more attention to how their body feels may be more prone to anxiety as well as to PGAD.

Doctors and scientists are currently researching effective treatments for PGAD. In one study, physical therapy exercises were found to be helpful. For some women, masturbation to orgasm helps. Other times, women find that applying an ice pack to their genitals helps relieve the feelings of genital pressure or arousal. Women who experience a great deal of anxiety, shame, or embarrassment about their genital arousal symptoms may be helped by meeting with a sex therapist—again, while PGAD isn't "all in their heads," counseling or therapy can be helpful in aiding women to relax and focus on things other than their bodily sensations (which may exacerbate their discomfort).

If a woman's symptoms started after she began taking a certain medication, she should mention this to her health care provider, as there may be another medication or another type of treatment available without such side effects. And while a minority of patients with PGAD felt that their symptoms started while they were taking SSRI antidepressants, a larger number of these patients have felt that their symptoms improved while taking antidepressants.

If you experience PGAD, please know that there is reason to be hopeful that your condition can be treated so you can feel better and more comfortable in your body. If your health care provider isn't knowledgeable on the topic, try to find a doctor in your community who specializes in sexual medicine (see Resources) or bring your health care provider copies of some of the research articles listed in the back of the book so that they can become familiar with PGAD and help you to manage it effectively. Consider, too, whether it's possible to reframe your situation. Although some women are bothered by feelings of constant arousal, others are not. Might there be a way to look at your situation from a different perspective?

6. What to do if . . . you experience vaginal dryness even though you're too young for menopause

Vaginal dryness typically kicks in on a more regular basis as women approach menopause (commonly in their mid-to-late forties or early fifties, although some women reach menopause at younger or older ages). However, there are a number of reasons why even younger women may experience vaginal dryness. In our recent National Survey of Sexual Health and Behavior, my research team found that about one-third of American women (even very young women) report having experienced vaginal lubrication difficulties during their most recent sex act.[15] More specifically, 35 percent of women ages eighteen to twenty-four reported lubrication difficulties during the most recent time they had sex as did 28 percent of women ages twenty-five to twenty-nine, 31 percent of women in their thirties, 36 percent of women in their forties, and nearly half of women in their fifties. This is striking. It suggests a few things to me. Perhaps many young women and their partners are rushing into sex without adequate foreplay.

Or the sex they are often having lasts a long time, or is quite vigorous and rough, thus drying the vagina. Or Mother Nature built the vagina to make enough lubrication to be "sufficient" for sex that is kind of, sort of comfortable, but that "works," and if we want sex to be wetter, we have to take matters into our own hands through foreplay and store-bought lubricants.

Insufficient vaginal lubrication is different from vaginal dryness. Not having enough vaginal lubrication can happen to any woman and is more often a result of rushing into sex without much foreplay, having sex after a shower or bath (warm water dries the vagina out), or having a tight genital fit (for example, if your partner or sex toy is very big, or your vagina is quite small).

Vaginal dryness is a whole different ball game. It's more chronic and ongoing and is typically caused by low levels of estrogen. Remember: estrogen plays an important role in producing vaginal lubrication. This is why it's more common among postmenopausal women whose ovaries have stopped producing estrogens.

So which young women are candidates for ongoing vaginal dryness? Women who are breastfeeding, as their estrogen levels are typically low, may experience uncomfortable vaginal dryness. Also, women who have had their ovaries removed, for example as part of a hysterectomy or as part of surgical treatment for cancer, may experience vaginal dryness (this is sometimes called "surgical menopause," meaning that by surgically removing the hormone-producing ovaries, the woman has effectively gone into menopause). If your vagina feels uncomfortable, such as feeling dry or sandpaper-ish during sexual activities as well as daily activities, let your health care provider know. She or he may recommend a vaginal moisturizer that you can apply at home, and it can make a world of difference.

7. What to do if . . . sexual penetration is impossible (can't get it in)

This is another case for a vulvovaginal expert. It's also an instance in which you may want to connect with a sex therapist. Often, when women feel that they absolutely cannot go through with vaginal penetration or intercourse, there's a lot of fear and panic that surrounds the issue—and sometimes a good deal of strain on the relationship. A sex therapist who has experience treating women with vaginismus (a name for a condition that describes women who feel unable to experience vaginal penetration, often with a great deal of fear or anxiety, even though they want to and have tried to) or vulvodynia (unexplained vaginal pain) may be a helpful guide on your journey to getting better. A medical doctor or nurse is instrumental in checking to make sure that there are no health conditions causing the pain or difficulty with penetration. A therapist can be helpful in terms of coaching you (and your partner if you have one) through attempts you make at home, and in private, to have sex. Your doctor, nurse, or therapist may recommend the use of vaginal dilators (see sidebar on page 35).

8. What to do if . . . you "squirt" (female ejaculation)

You're in good company. Many women release significant amounts of fluid during sexual arousal or orgasm. This is sometimes called "female ejaculation," although not all sexual health professionals like or use this term because women's sexual fluids are not precisely the same as male ejaculate (semen).

Scientific research is lagging in this area so the percentage of women who experience female ejaculation is not known. What we do know is that the fluid comes out of the urethra, but if you're worried that you're peeing during sex, you can relax. Female ejaculation is not the same as urine (pee), and the chances of that are very, very low. Researchers who have conducted chemical analyses of female ejaculate have found that it is distinct from urine, and that it is composed of creatinine, prostate specific antigen, glucose, fructose, and other substances.[16-17]

That said, if you accidentally release urine when you laugh, cough, or sneeze, or if you have to pee so often throughout the day or night that it bothers you, let your health care provider know. In one study my research team conducted at Indiana University, we found that women's incontinence symptoms were among the biggest predictors of less pleasurable sex. If you can get your urinary concerns addressed and, if needed, treated, you may feel more confident in bed.

But back to female ejaculation: as far as scientists can tell, there is nothing unhealthy about this experience. It happens to millions of women.

Although it surprises some women and their partners at first, many grow to enjoy it as part of their sexual experience. I like to think of female ejaculation as a "beauty's in the eye of the beholder" kind of thing; some people aren't thrilled with female ejaculation, while others are. A friend of mine who often experiences female ejaculation looks to it as a sign of great sex. And a man I know who's come across it a few times says it's always a surprise when he encounters it, but he loves pleasing women so much that it's never a bad surprise. It just is what it is.

A few words about prep work: as with men's "wet spots," some women lay a towel down on the bed, or other sex surface, before they have sex to minimize the post-sex cleanup. Others just let it flow. It's totally up to you and your partner.

9. What to do if . . . your labia get pushed in during sex

Easy: pause for a moment during sex and pull them out. If one or both labia are pushed in in such a way that you need your male partner to pull out so you can remove them (rare, but possible), ask him to gently pull out for a moment. And before you go blaming your labia size for your discomfort, let me reassure you that labia of any shape or size can get pushed inside uncomfortably during sex. Labiaplasty (surgery to resize and reshape the labia) is definitely not a guarantee against this experience, as even women with itsy bitsy inner labia (less than one or two centimeters long) have this happen to them at times. Trust me on this one.

10. What to do if . . . your vagina tears during sex

I think of tearing during sex as falling into one of three categories. Each type is important and requires a different strategy.

The first kind of tearing is quite common and can be thought of as very tiny tears—invisible to the naked eye—that occur inside the vaginal canal or around the vaginal entrance. These tears are the result of friction between a woman's vagina and the penetrating fingers, penis, or sex toy. They're more likely to happen if a woman is not well lubricated during penetration (such as during sex in the shower, when her natural vaginal lubrication may have dried, making sex feel rough and uncomfortable).

These kinds of tears also sometimes happen if her male partner's penis is larger than average, or if sex is vigorous or rough or lasts a long time. If you experience this kind of vaginal tearing (and many of us have), you might not feel any pain or discomfort during sex. Later on, however, when you go to the bathroom, you might notice a small amount of light-colored blood on the toilet paper after you wipe yourself, or you might notice a trace of blood on your underwear. This has certainly happened to me before, and spending more time in foreplay or using a water-based lubricant has done the trick for me. This kind of vaginal tearing is usually not serious and often heals on its own within two to four days, particularly if you avoid sex or masturbation while it heals. If you repeatedly experience this kind of vaginal tearing, try using a water-based lubricant during sex to see if this reduces the frequency of tearing. You might also mention it to your health care provider, as sometimes there are health reasons (such as low levels of estrogen) for women being prone to vaginal tearing.

A second kind of tearing isn't in the vagina, but on the vulva. These are also very small tears that you might not be able to see with the naked eye; they're just differently placed. Instead of being inside the vaginal canal, they may be on the vestibule (the area around the vaginal entrance), the labia, or just below the vaginal entrance. If you repeatedly experience pain, discomfort, or bleeding on your genital skin, let your health care provider know. Some skin conditions, including one called lichen sclerosus, can make a woman's genital skin more vulnerable to tearing during masturbation or sex with a partner. Treating the skin condition, such as with a cream prescribed by a doctor, can strengthen the skin and reduce the risk of tearing. Women who are breastfeeding or in menopause, or who otherwise have low levels of estrogen, may also be more prone to vulvar tearing. Again, this is something that should be brought to your health care provider's attention.

The third and most serious type of tearing during sex is an accidental tear or injury. Sometimes women tear pretty badly during sex. This can result in significant pain and can be noticeably bloody. If this happens to you, call your health care provider immediately and/or go to the emergency room. Sometimes the cut can be treated at home. However, your health care provider may recommend that you use a prescription antibiotic cream or ointment to reduce the risk of infection (after all, the vagina and vulva are close to the anus, so there's some risk of getting bacteria near the cut). Other times, genital cuts are severe enough that they require stitches and other kinds of medical treatment. I once experienced a sex cut from vaginal intercourse and it was certainly no picnic (having my boyfriend at the time put on his glasses and inspect my vagina under full bright lights was also no picnic, but it gave us something to laugh about later). However, I was fortunate that my health care provider felt I didn't need to come in to the office or get stitches. Based on our conversation on the phone, she felt the cut sounded small and shallow enough that I could treat it at home with a prescription antibiotic ointment. That said, I've had friends and students who have had more severe cuts that required trips to the emergency room and stitches. It's not your fault if you get a sex cut and if you do, don't let embarrassment get in the way of getting good health care. Always do your best to take care of your vulva (and the rest of your body too).

11. What to do if . . . you notice a lump down there

Many genital lumps and bumps are completely harmless (such as moles or other natural skin bumps) and are benign, meaning not cancerous (read *The V Book: A Doctor's Guide to Complete Vulvovaginal Health* for an entire chapter on the many lumps and bumps that occur on women's genitals). Some are moles. Other lumps and bumps are the result of infected hair follicles, or are genital warts caused by certain strains of the human papillomavirus (HPV).

In rare cases, however, a lump or bump on the genitals may be a sign of cancer, which is more effectively treated with higher survival rates when detected early. It's better to be safe than sorry and tell your health care providers about your new discoveries down there rather than keeping them to yourself. Sometimes women notice other sorts of genital changes, such as an enlarged clitoris, that may be a sign of other health problems, including some cancers. Remember: all genital changes should be mentioned to your health care provider. And if you feel that your questions or concerns aren't being addressed by that person, switch doctors or get a second opinion.

Most women will never get vulvar cancer. However, it's always a good idea to become more familiar with your body, and it is possible that you may notice other important health issues through practicing VSE, so grab your mirror (and your lovely vulva!) and start looking.

Sex Smarts Quiz

1. The process of checking out one's mons, clitoris, labia, and other neighboring areas about once each month is called
   a. Vaginal self-examination
   b. Cervical self-examination
   c. Vulvar self-examination
   d. Breast self-examination
2. Women who feel bothered by a sense of genital arousal that won't go away (even after masturbation or sex to the point of orgasm) may be experiencing
   a. Persistent Genital Arousal Disorder
   b. Labiaplasty
   c. Labia puff procedure
   d. Vaginal dryness
3. The Great Wall of Vagina is
   a. A chorus of women who sing pro-vagina songs
   b. An art project aimed at celebrating the diversity of women's genitals
   c. A series of long, impressive stone walls located in China
   d. None of the above

Answers
   1. c
   2. a
   3. b

CHAPTER 2

The Penis and Beyond: His Magical, Mysterious Places of Wonder

We already know how I feel about genitals being incredible places of potential for joy, excitement, orgasms, and wonder. But men's genitals, which are foreign to women, can also be confusing, frustrating places of blunder. It's common for women who partner with men to have a very real need for information about men's genitals, including how to touch them, lick them, have sex with them, the differences in circumcised versus uncircumcised penises, and more.

In the many years I've worked as a sex educator at the Kinsey Institute and a sex columnist for various magazines, I've received thousands of questions about men's genitals. Some of the more common questions include

• Is an uncircumcised penis as clean as a circumcised one?
• Can I get pregnant from his pre-cum?
• Is it possible to be allergic to a man's semen?
• What should I do if I get semen in my eyes?
• Can a penis actually break?

By the end of this chapter, you will have answers to these questions and will understand a whole host of things related to men's bodies that can make for better, easier, more pleasurable sex. You might even teach the men in your life a few things.

PENIS PARTS—INSIDE AND OUT!

As you can see in the diagram opposite, the bottom of the penis (the base) is where the shaft meets the pubic area. The shaft changes the most in size during arousal. Sometimes, men are called "showers" if their penis doesn't grow too much when they become erect; these penises are the original WYSIWYG body parts ("what you see is what you get"). Growers, on the other hand, expand significantly in length and circumference when they become sexually excited, aroused, and erect. Because some men are showers and others are growers, there is no way to tell from looking at a man's flaccid (soft) penile state how big or small his penis will be when it's erect. Locker rooms only reveal so much—or, rather, so little.

The glans penis is the science-speak name for the head of the penis. On the underside of the penis is the frenulum, the triangular area of skin that connects just below the glans. The frenulum is a sensitive area for many men. You might try touching, licking, or kissing this area during sex play or oral sex with a partner to see whether your partner enjoys it or finds it adds an extra bit of excitement to his experience.

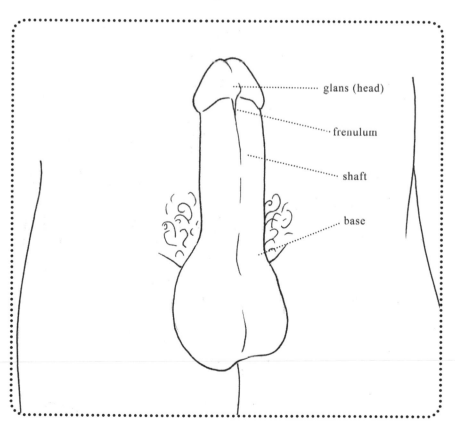

THE SPECTRUM OF SIZE

Many men have anxieties about the size of their flaccid (soft) or erect (hard) penis. For some men, childhood or teenage teasing can make them feel self-conscious about their penis size well into adulthood. And it's not only guys with smaller penis sizes that may have borne the cruel brunt of teasing; many men with larger penises recall having been teased as teenagers. I've heard from men who feel ashamed and embarrassed to have been called names like "elephant cock" or "moose dick" when growing up, or to have had their genitals compared to sausages. If you grew up with a little brother, raised sons, or taught or babysat boys, then you likely know that boys are often just as sensitive to teasing as girls are; the main difference is that they learn early on that it's not "manly" to show their sensitivity and, consequently, they hide their hurt feelings. Of course, hiding embarrassment only buries it deeper, which means that there are millions, if not billions, of adult men in the world who might feel badly about their penises.

Outright teasing and name-calling aren't the only things that make men feel badly about their bodies. Some men have removed their pants to get ready for sex with someone new, only to notice a disappointed or worried look on their partner's face as she or he spotted their extra-large (or extra-small) penis. It can be difficult for men not to take these shocked looks or high school teasing to heart, so be gentle with the male sex partner(s) in your life. Try to give your partner props when it comes to their penis without making it sound like you're doing it only to be nice. Compliment him on his penis by saying things like "I love how well you fit inside me" or "There's little I love more than feeling your penis/cock/dick in my hands" (everyone has different comfort levels and preferences when it comes to genital names, so use a word that feels comfortable or sexy to you and your partner).

HIS SIZE: WHAT'S NORMAL?

One of the most common questions we've received at the Kinsey Institute since we first opened our doors has to do with penis size. Many men want to know how they measure up. In the early-to mid-twentieth century, Dr. Alfred Kinsey asked men to measure their penises and send their measurements back to him, which resulted in some of the earliest data collected about the wide range of penis sizes.[1] Over the years, scientists and men's magazines alike have explored the question, as have people in the privacy of their own bedrooms. So what's average?

A 2006 study published in *Psychology of Men & Masculinity* found that the average erect penis length was 5.3 inches long (13.5 cm) and more than two-thirds of men (68 percent) measured between 4.6 and 6.0 inches (11.7 cm and 15.2 cm, respectively).[2] Only 2.5 percent of men had a penis size that was longer than 6.9 inches (17.5 cm) and only 2.5 percent measured less than 3.7 inches (9.4 cm).

Aside from size, there are also issues of bend and curvature. Many men have a natural bend to their penis. Some men use this to their advantage by using their bend or curve to massage the front wall of a woman's vagina (her "G Spot" area). In most cases, the bend or curve isn't an issue. However, if a bend or curve appears to become more extreme, if it's angled so sharply that it makes intercourse difficult, or if there's discomfort or pain associated with it, a man should check in with his health care provider.

Manscaping

Over the past decade, an increasing number of men have been grooming their body hair. Some salons specialize in what they call a man's "back, sack, and crack," referring to his back, his scrotum, and in between his butt cheeks. One of the most common pubic hair removal methods for men is trimming with scissors. If done sober, wide-awake, and not in the middle of an earthquake, there is little risk of accidental cuts. Some men shave some of the hair on their pubic mound or penis, although the closer one gets to the penis or scrotum, the more careful one should be so as to avoid accidental nicks or cuts. Some men choose to go to a salon and get waxed by a professional, but some salons refuse to wax men's genitals, even though it's common for salons to offer full Brazilian waxes to women. If a man you know is interested in waxing, he should call around to find a salon that has an experienced aes-thetician on staff who routinely waxes men's genitals; this is not a job for an amateur.

A River Runs Through It

Inside the penis is where the magic begins. There are three chambers of spongy tissue, two of which are made of spongy erectile tissue (the cor-pora cavernosa). The third chamber is also spongy, but the urethra—the tube that carries urine and semen out of the body—runs through it. Knowing about these parts is essential to understanding men's erections. Here's how they happen:

When a man becomes sexually excited, either from physical touching of his penis or from thinking exciting thoughts, more blood flows to his genitals. Remember: this happens with women too. The difference is that for men, the arteries inside the three spongy chambers fill up and as they enlarge, they press against narrow veins inside the penis, making it more difficult for blood to leave the penis. This leads to more blood flowing into the penis than out, which is what makes an erection. We'll talk in greater detail about erections—including the various forces that shape erections and what to do when they falter—in a later chapter.

A Cut Above the Rest?
Foreskin and Circumcision

In certain parts of the world, including the US, many male infants undergo circumcision (removal of the foreskin) because of their fam-ily's religious or cultural beliefs. The World Health Organization estimates that about 30 percent of males have been circumcised, typically as infants, children, or adolescents.[3] When male circumcision is performed during adulthood, it is usually for medical reasons, such as if a man has dif-ficulty or pain retracting his foreskin.

Some groups advocate making male circumcision illegal, just as female genital circumcision (which can involve varying degrees of cutting or removal of the labia, clitoris, and other vulva parts) is illegal in many parts of the world. However, an increasing number of studies have shown that men who have been circumcised have a lower risk of contracting STIs and HIV.[4-5] As a result, some health groups now recommend routine male circumcision in countries with high HIV prevalence. Other scientists are against this policy, given that it is ultimately people's behaviors—what they do—that put them at risk of HIV, not only whether or not they have foreskin.

For example, if a man uses condoms consistently and correctly when he has sex with a partner, he is unlikely to get most STIs or HIV. Another way to prevent STIs and HIV is to only have sex with an uninfected partner in a monogamous relationship. In other words, there is a great deal that can be done to reduce one's risk of STIs and HIV that has nothing to do with whether or not a man has a foreskin. And as some activists point out, it is unlikely that people would ever suggest a policy to promote female genital circumcision even if it were found to be true that the practice resulted in a lower STI or HIV infection rate for women.

What do you think? Should boys and girls be treated the same or differently when it comes to genital circumcision? Should there be the same level of protections for male infants and children worldwide as there is for female infants and children? In what ways do you feel that male circumcision and female circumcision procedures are similar or different?

CIRCUMCISION AND SEX

A common question people have about male circumcision has to do with sex. I get a lot of questions about the cleanliness of men's circumcised versus uncircumcised penises (especially in relation to oral sex); I also get a lot of questions about whether women who have sex with men should use different sexual techniques for uncircumcised versus circumcised partners.

Strikingly little is known about how male circumcision affects sex for men or their partners. Some studies of men who were circumcised as adults suggest that circumcision is linked to decreased penile sensation. This isn't always a bad thing, as some men feel that the reduced sensation helps them last longer during sex. Other men who were circumcised as infants as a result of a decision made by their doctor or parents before they were old enough to give consent feel upset that they were not given the choice to make themselves. They will never know if they would have had different penile sensation, or better (or worse) sex, if they still had their foreskin.

Then there's the issue of a man's partner. One interesting study published in the *British Journal of Urology* found that women who had had sex with both circumcised and uncircumcised men reported a greater likelihood of orgasm, as well as multiple orgasm, with an uncircumcised partner.[6] Sex with uncircumcised men was also judged to have lasted longer as compared to sex with circumcised men. However, this was a small study and I'm not aware of any others like it, so it's difficult to know how valid these results are.

The first time I dated a man who was uncircumcised, I felt slightly nervous as things progressed. Even though I knew that circumcision was not a matter of hygiene (it's clear from medical opinion that both cut and uncut men are "clean"), I had questions. What would sex feel like with an uncircumcised man? And would condom use be trickier, given that research has found that condoms sometimes slip off more often on uncircumcised men?[7] What I ultimately found is that I love penises with or without foreskin. More than that, I was surprised to find that once my partner and I stopped using condoms, I could feel his foreskin move along my vaginal walls during sex. It was a new sensation to me and a wonderful one, and I had seen nothing written about it previously in sex research articles. I couldn't feel it all of the time, but I did sometimes, and it felt nice. Feeling his foreskin also seemed to make it easier to experience orgasm during vaginal intercourse with him and again with a subsequent partner who was uncircumcised. Can I guarantee that you'll have a similar experience? Of course not. But you might have fun trying.

FRIENDS WITH BENEFITS: THE BOYS

Now let's turn our attention to the penis's closest "friends": namely, the scrotum and its inside parts. The scrotum is the outside package. It houses the testicles and other parts, such as the epididymis, which sits over each testicle and plays a role in sperm production. By keeping the testicles hung away from a man's trunk, they stay cooler, which helps keep sperm production running smoothly. Down the middle of the scrotum, you may notice something that looks like a line or a ridge of skin, called the "raphe." This is a normal part of men's genitals and is essentially the "seam" where tissues met up together and fused while in the womb. Pretty cool, huh?

But let's get back to men's testicles: if you have yet to feel them, check them out on a willing and interested partner. Men's testicles are egg shaped and can be felt from all angles, even turned around gently in one's fingers (some men don't like this, so ask first). Some men have highly sensitive testicles and don't want to be touched, licked, or sucked there, whereas others love it when their partner pays attention to their testicles. Ask your partner what he likes before getting too eagerly involved down there. Between the back of the scrotum and the anus is the perineum, casually called the "taint" (as in "t'aint the balls, t'aint the butt") or "tween" (as it's *between* these two parts).

Teabagging

Get your mind out of the kitchen and into the bedroom. When used as a sex term, "teabagging" refers to taking a man's testicle into one's mouth. Some men "teabag" their partner, which may go something like this: his partner is lying down on the bed, mouth open, and then he squats on top of her and lowers his testicle into her waiting mouth for oral stimulation—kind of like how a teabag is lowered into a cup of hot water.

That's What (Se)men Are Made Of

Semen (also called ejaculate) is a combination of fluids from several different body parts including the seminal vesicles and the prostate gland. Sperm make up only a tiny amount of seminal volume. A small amount of fluid is from the Cowper's glands, which are small, pea-sized glands at the base of the penis. The Cowper's glands secrete fluid that may begin dripping out of the urethra long before a man actually ejaculates any semen. As it comes out first, it's called "pre-ejaculate" (or pre-cum). It does not contain sperm. Sometimes the pre-ejaculate doesn't make it all the way out of the penis ahead of time and the fluids end up getting swept up with the other seminal fluids, completely unnoticed.

Pre-ejaculate is one of the things I find most fascinating about men's bodies. This small amount of fluid plays two important roles. By being released first, the fluid helps lubricate a man's penis and, during intercourse with a woman, helps to lubricate the vagina. Also, pre-ejaculate helps to make the man's urethra less acidic so that by the time the sperm come out during ejaculation, they survive the trip out of the penis. If the urethra were too acidic, the sperm might be damaged. Pre-ejaculate helps sperm stay safe.

The Prostate

The prostate gland sits beneath a man's bladder. Although small, it produces about 25 to 30 percent of the volume of semen. That may not seem like a lot, but some men are pretty active in terms of their masturbation or partnered sex lives and may keep their prostate quite busy. This is completely fine as far as the prostate is concerned. In fact, some research suggests that frequent masturbation or sex while men are young (in their twenties and thirties) is linked to a lower risk of prostate cancer in older age.[8] Instead of making fun of a man or scolding him for frequent masturbation, why not encourage it, take part in it, or keep the house stocked with tissues or sufficient "bad towels" (unless you want him to use the good ones, which I wouldn't advise lest they lose their softness)?

As men get into their forties and fifties, it is common for the prostate to enlarge, which can make some men feel as though they have to urinate (pee) even when they don't (older age brings lots of these "false alarms"). This may feel like sweet justice to all the moms who spent their twenties, thirties, or forties running to the bathroom while they were pregnant or after they had their baby while their partner hung out on the couch or stayed asleep in bed. Frequent urination should always be brought to the attention of one's health care provider.

Of course, other things can go wrong with the prostate that are far more serious. Prostate cancer is, unfortunately, one of the most common cancers among men as they age. Men should be encouraged to check in with their health care providers for information about annual prostate exams as they get into their forties and fifties (recommendations will vary from man to man depending on their personal health and family history).

—Making It Easy—

12. What to do if . . . he's anxious about his penis size

Although size seems to matter to some sex partners, the differences among most men's penis size are so minor that it matters less than many think. This is especially true given what we talked about in the last chapter: that the vagina changes in shape and size during sexual arousal and depending on the sexual position. Vaginal lubrication and store-bought lubricants can also change the way sex feels, as can a person's psychological excitement or how "into" sex they feel. If you think back to your earliest sexual experiences, you can probably recall times when you didn't have intercourse or any other kind of contact with a penis, but kissing, making out, and touching each other were so incredibly arousing that you thought you might burst with excitement. To focus on penis size as the most important thing to sex is to miss the point—and a whole host of other ways you could be making sex better.

Some men, feeling anxious about their penis size, might ask, "Am I big enough for you?" or "How do I compare to other guys you've been with?" These are tricky questions. Size matters less than many people—including many experienced women—think it does. If a woman's vagina is very wet and lubricated, her vagina may feel roomier or he will feel smaller (it all depends on your perspective). Then again, if her vagina is less well lubricated, it may feel tighter and his penis may seem larger or as if there is more sensation during sex. This is one reason why sex between men and women is rarely about one person's size and more about genital fit between the two people.

That said, there are only so many ways to help a guy feel good about his penis. And while you can be helpful and encouraging, it's not your job to stroke his ego, or his penis's ego. But you can help. Here's what I suggest:

If his penis has even the smallest chance of working for you, then fall in love with it. Kiss it, stroke it, and look at it with enthusiasm during oral sex. Tell him that one day you'd be happy to sit around, stream a movie, and make out and lick his penis—assuming, of course, that this is true and you've been tested for STIs and are comfortable with each other's STI status. Tell him how good it feels inside you or how great you two fit together. Squeeze your vaginal muscles around it. Slide up and down his penis during woman-on-top sex. Get the picture? Make his penis a wonderful part of sex play.

If he asks you to compare his penis size to other men, tell him that his penis is a good size for you and that you refuse to compare. Let him know, too, that size is only part of the picture. All the other things matter, too, such as _____. Fill in the blanks with what matters to you, such as oral sex technique, being romantic in bed, getting into dirty talk, being open to bondage play, using sex toys together, or having a penchant for public sex; this is your chance to reinforce what's important to you. Bottom line—*show* him that his penis is an amazing part of sex and you won't have to keep *telling* him.

13. What to do if . . . he's achingly big

If your partner's penis is uncomfortably large, don't give up! This is easier to tackle than it may seem. Try these things before cutting him loose—I know a few wonderful couples these tricks have worked for who were able to stay together even though they initially thought they weren't a good fit.

- **Check in with your health care provider.** You need to make sure that all is OK on your end. Some women have anatomical issues such as a hymenal ring that prevents entry. Other times, pain disorders such as vulvodynia or vaginismus are at the root of what feels like impossible entry.

• **Spend at least fifteen minutes in foreplay.** Do things that you truly find exciting and arousing. This may take some courage if you haven't previously let him know what drives you wild. One sex therapist I know advises women to delay having sex until their vagina is practically throbbing with arousal and anticipation. Foreplay gives your body time to lubricate naturally and also kick-starts the wondrous process of vaginal tenting (this is when the vagina—which is normally about three to four inches long when unaroused—grows in length and width when a woman is aroused; vaginal tenting can lead to more comfortable and pleasurable intercourse).

• **Play with a vibrator.** Vibration stimulates both men's and women's sexual response. In a study my research team at Indiana University published in 2009 in the *Journal of Sexual Medicine,* we found that vibrator use was linked to greater arousal, ease of orgasm, and lubrication. Several minutes of vibrator play may help with vaginal lubrication and tenting, which can make a larger penis size a more comfortable fit.

• **Lube it up!** If you're not currently trying to become pregnant (lubricant can interfere with sperm movement), try adding lubricant to your or his genitals before sex begins. Start with a dime- or nickel-sized amount of a water-based lubricant and add more as wanted. Lube can be particularly helpful for accommodating men with thick penises.

• **Share the load.** Get a soft, flexible masturbation sleeve (also called a pocket pussy) that has a hole on each end, available from many in-home sex toy party companies, sex boutiques, and websites. Lubricate the sleeve, slide it down his shaft, and hop on top (don't literally hop on top of his penis, it's just an expression; but do get on top position-wise). If his penis is extra long, this can be a true sex-saver because it means the sleeve will squeeze the bottom three to six inches of his shaft while you stimulate the rest by being on top. He gets penile stimulation and you get comfort. Win-win.

• **Reach out.** He might find it helpful to connect with The Large Penis Support Group (www.lpsg.org), where members provide support and tips (including sex tips) on message boards.

14. What to do if . . . he's too small for the job

Don't despair! Here's what to do:

• **Keep a towel nearby** to dab your genitals and his when things get wet and lubricated. By drying them slightly, you can increase the friction to heighten sensitivity for both of you.

• **Insert a tampon into your vagina before sex.** Let it soak up your vaginal wetness for about thirty seconds or a minute, then remove it and proceed as usual. By slightly drying your vagina, you will likely feel more sensation.

• **Expand your perspective.** If you've never really gotten into oral sex, sex toy play, finger play, BDSM (bondage, domination, submission, masochism, etc.), or threesomes, this may be your chance. If you're really into a smaller-sized guy and his penis size isn't doing it for you, see what else brings you pleasure. And try to not feel as if you're settling: there are many reasons we find ourselves looking into things we least expected for pleasure. After all, the only reason I ever first learned to orgasm during vaginal intercourse is because I was dating someone with rapid ejaculation. The oral sex was only so-so (through no fault of his own; I hadn't put much effort into communicating with him what I liked), and I ended up learning to experience orgasm during intercourse in a desperate attempt to have orgasms when we had sex. I learned to do it quickly too! Although my partner's penis size was larger than average, I see no reason why you couldn't take a similar approach to sex with a smaller than average-sized partner. If your partner's small size is a downer, maybe you can make another part of sex (like oral sex) more awesome and size won't matter as much.

• **Consider medical help.** This isn't for everyone, but a very small percent of men have what's called micropenis and in this case a surgical procedure can help to elongate the penis. However, penile surgeries carry risks of complications, including the development of scar tissue and painful erections, so he'd be wise to check in with an experienced surgeon or two before deciding to go this route.

• **Check into penile extenders.** Sex toys have grown increasingly sophisticated over the past decade. There are more penile extenders on the market than ever before that are high quality, that aren't awkward during sex, and that can be fun for the guy wearing it as well as the partner on the receiving end. Just make sure to lube it up before use.

15. What to do if . . . his penis is highly sensitive

The glans is the most sensitive part of a man's penis. The embryonic tissue that develops into the clitoris for females is the same tissue that develops into the glans penis for males. This explains why the glans is as sensitive as it is; after all, they come from the same tissue with the same number of nerve endings, except the nerve endings in the clitoris are more concentrated.

This has its pros and cons. The fact that the glans is so sensitive means that men can often experience orgasm fairly easily during intercourse or masturbation—much more easily than many women can, as the glans gets lots of direct stimulation during sex. However, the sensitive nature of the glans means that some men feel overly sensitive and may either back away from stimulation, especially after sex, or feel highly stimulated to the point where they ejaculate more quickly than they'd like.

Just as some women can only take so much clitoral stimulation before they feel it's too much and they need a breather, some men feel similarly. Some guys enjoy stimulation of their glans right up until they ejaculate.

Then, it's hands-off and mouth-off. If your partner has a very sensitive penis, give him some breathing room post-ejaculation. Stay involved in the sex act by kissing him or stimulating the base of his penis, his scrotum, or perineum until he's finished ejaculating, then give him some space.

16. What to do if . . . his penis "pops" during sex

If you are ever having sex with a man and you hear a popping or snapping sound or he grabs his penis out of pain, try to get him to go to the emergency room. After all, a penis can "break." (Sort of.) As the spongy chambers fill with blood, they become stiff, and the lining around them (called the tunica albuginea) is only flexible up to a point, at which the penile fracture occurs. If a man is having vigorous sex and is thrusting in and out, or his partner is hopping up and down on top, his penis may come out of and accidentally hit against his partner's body rather than going back inside the vagina or anus from whence it came. Early treatment—often involving draining blood from the penis—is important. If left untreated, swelling and infection may develop, as might scar tissue (which can result in the penis forming a bend or curve), or it can result in painful erections. It's nothing to feel embarrassed about, as it does happen sometimes; US data from 2006 to 2007 show 1,043 cases of penile fracture, more than a third of which occurred over the weekend when people may be more likely to have sex.[10] Penile fracture may also be more likely to happen to younger men— the average age of patients was 36.7 years—and those with strong erections, as there needs to be some degree of rigidity for it to break in the first place. (A softer penis would be more likely to simply bend.) Yet another study, published in 2011, found that an unusually high number of penile fractures happened to men while they were having affairs and having sex outside the bedroom (e.g., in a car, elevator, office).[11] The take-home message here is that a popping sound from a penis necessitates a trip to the doctor. Stat.

17. What to do if . . . his penis is pierced

As fancy as penises are, some people want to make them even fancier by way of piercing, which dates at least as far back as the *Kama Sutra*. Men may get pierced on their pubic mound, glans penis, mid-shaft of the penis, on the scrotum, or along the frenulum (the underside of the penis). Some piercings heal quickly; the Prince Albert style (one of the more common styles among the pierced), for example, can take as little as two to four weeks to heal. This piercing goes through the top of the urethra and out the glans (head), and some men feel that it offers urethral stimulation during masturbation or sex. Although genital piercings are thought to enhance sexual sensation, there has been so little scientific research on genital piercing that it's not known whether this is true for most people.

Some people will tell you that genital piercings don't cause problems and often this is true. However, genital piercings have been linked to a greater risk of STI infection, as even long after piercing there may be a chronic, low level of irritation around the piercing, making STIs easier to pass. There are other things to consider too. Some people's piercings hurt their partner during sex, such as by causing trauma or irritation to the vagina or anus. During oral sex, some people have choked on their partner's piercing, chipped their teeth, or even trapped a piercing between their teeth.[11] Genital piercings can also cause condoms to tear. If your partner has a piercing and you are willing to have sex with him or her anyway, or are excited and feel into it, tread carefully. Get tested for STIs and HIV together and make sure that you are comfortable with each other's STI and HIV status, as condoms may not be practical or as effective for you two (although they're worth a shot anyway). You might also want to start with gentle sex until you get used to how sex feels with a pierced partner.

18. What to do if . . . he's uncircumcised and you want to use condoms

Condoms can be trickier to use on uncircumcised men. Condoms sometimes slip off uncircumcised men's penises more often than they slip off men who have been circumcised, probably because of the way the foreskin slips and slides over the penis (perhaps pushing the condom). Roomier condoms, such as those that are looser along the shaft, may be good choices for men with foreskins. Whatever you choose, make sure that your partner's penis is fully erect and that his foreskin is retracted before putting the condom on and rolling it all the way down to the base. He should pay attention to how it feels during sex and stop to readjust if he notices slippage. Finally, like any man (circumcised or not), he should hold on to the base of the condom when withdrawing his penis from his partner's vagina, anus, or mouth. Try not to let a man's uncircumcised penis get in the way of safer, pleasurable sex because it absolutely doesn't have to. Sex can be great with a man whether he's circumcised or not.

A Handy Tip

One of the most important bits of information I've learned from dating uncircumcised men, as well as from receiving emails and letters from uncircumcised male readers of my sex columns, is that their foreskin can be quite sensitive during manual stimulation (hand jobs). Some uncircumcised men say that it can be uncomfortable or even hurt if their foreskin is pushed down too much during hand jobs, so you might want to start out gently or at least pay attention to your partner's response while using your hands to pleasure him.

19. What to do if . . . it hurts for him to retract his foreskin

Easy decision: he should mention this to a health care provider. There is nothing you should be doing at home on your own for this one. There are some skin conditions that can cause inflammation of a man's skin and other issues that can lead to difficulty or pain when retracting his foreskin. Sometimes health care providers are able to prescribe topical creams to treat the condition; other times, circumcision is recommended. Certainly there may be instances when an uncircumcised man's partner pulls too hard on his foreskin, such as during hand jobs (see sidebar). But if it hurts for his foreskin to retract, whether during masturbation or partnered sex, and no matter how gently he tries to retract it, that's another issue and it deserves attention from a professional.

20. What to do if . . . his scrotum is sore

Encourage him to see a health care provider. A man's scrotum or testicles may feel sore or achy because of an infection or inflammation of his epididymis or other internal reproductive parts, and he may require treatment (sometimes via prescription antibiotics). If his doctor says there's nothing wrong, encourage him to get a second opinion, possibly from a urologist, as some men may have infections that aren't regularly tested for in most clinics.

21. What to do if . . . he finds a bump on one of his testicles

All testicular lumps and bumps and soreness should be checked out by a health care provider. Testicular cancer may be diagnosed among men of all ages; however, it's more common among younger men. As teenagers, young men should learn to perform testicular self-examination and should continue to do so throughout adulthood. Some men even teach their partners to examine their testicles and they make this part of their shared sex play.

22. What to do if . . . he's curious about prostate play

The most common type of prostate play between men and women is done externally, without putting anything into the anus. You can stimulate his prostate by pressing your knuckles or fingers against his perineum during oral sex or vaginal sex. Start pressing the skin close to the scrotum, then work your way closer to his anal opening as you explore.

Though less commonly done between men and women, one can also stimulate a man's prostate internally with fingers or a sex toy (such as a butt plug or strap-on). As the anus doesn't lubricate naturally, you'd be wise to use plenty of water-based lubricant for internal prostate play. Slip a condom or a latex glove over anything (e.g., fingers, a sex toy, etc.) that goes into his anus and rectum to reduce the risk of transmitting infections or causing other kinds of damage. For finger play, wear a latex glove. For sex toy play, use a latex condom. If you two are new to this, start small, slowly and gently, paying attention to how he responds and if it hurts. Prostate play shouldn't hurt so if it does, stop. Also, avoid using anal desensitizers that may mask his discomfort or pain, which would be cues to stop. Finally, check out an anal-focused book such as one I wrote called *The Good in Bed Guide to Anal Pleasuring* (www.goodinbed.com) for more details, tips, and techniques.

23. What to do if . . . you think you're allergic to his semen

Some women are hypersensitive or allergic to semen.[12-13] Sometimes a woman reacts only to the semen of one particular man. Other times, she may react to semen from every man with whom she's had unprotected sex. If you have allergies, ask your partner if he's ingested any of the things you're allergic to, such as nuts, penicillin, or eggs. If so, he may be able to cut a food that you're allergic to out of his diet for your benefit. However, you should always check in with a health care provider if you notice an allergic reaction to semen, such as hives or difficulty breathing—and seek emergency medical care if this or other serious symptoms happen to you. Using a condom during sex can prevent a man's semen from coming into contact with his partner, which can help. Other couples look into treatment, which is becoming increasingly possible thanks to research by doctors who specialize in allergies and sensitivities. Check in with an allergy specialist or other health care provider if you suspect you might be hypersensitive or allergic to semen.

24. What to do if . . . his semen tastes terrible

There hasn't been any scientific study on how one can improve the taste of semen; however, some people believe that eating sweet, watery fruits such as pineapple or kiwi may help. Kiwi can be pricy to buy; however, pineapple is often available canned so it may be a more affordable and accessible option. As smell and taste are so interconnected, showering regularly and basic hygiene go a long way toward making oral sex more palatable. And if you don't like how it tastes, don't swallow: have him come in his or your hands or in a towel, or spit it out. You should never do something sexual that you don't want to do. But if you're open-minded about it and willing, it could be a pleasurable part of sex play for him—and perhaps he'll be willing to return the favor by being open and willing to try some of your ideas too.

25. What to do if . . . he gets pre-ejaculate near your vagina and you don't want to get pregnant

Pre-ejaculate (pre-cum) does not contain sperm, [14] which may be why withdrawal (the pulling-out method) is a decently effective method of birth control.[15] It's not a perfect method, as many men try to pull out in time but don't, and they end up ejaculating in or near their partner's vagina. That said, if a man ejaculates and then he and his partner start having sex soon after he ejaculates, and he doesn't pee in between, his urethra may have sperm hanging out in it. Then, if intercourse has begun when his Cowper's glands release pre-ejaculate the next time, those fluids may pick up the left-over sperm and carry them out of the penis and into the vagina. And in that case, pre-ejaculate could contain leftover sperm and may lead to a pregnancy.

My advice? If you don't want to become pregnant, use condoms and/or consider highly effective methods of birth control such as the birth control pill, shot, patch, or ring. And if you accidentally get pre-ejaculate in or near the vagina, chances are extremely low that you could become pregnant from that. If you're super worried about pregnancy, consider emergency contraception (the morning-after pill)—and take better precautions the next time.

26. What to do if . . . semen gets in your eye

Don't panic! Semen in one's eye isn't likely to cause blindness, but it might sting badly. You may find it helpful to splash lukewarm water on your eyes to help get the semen out. Your eyes may be pink and feel irritated for hours or into the next day. If you normally wear contacts, you might be more comfortable wearing glasses until your eyes feel better. If you're not sure of your partner's STI status, or if you're concerned that he might have chlamydia, gonorrhea, syphilis, or HIV, tell your health care provider what happened; you may need to be tested for STIs and may benefit from an eye exam. Pubic lice (crabs) may take up residence in your eyelashes if you perform oral sex on a man who has pubic lice and whose hairs get awfully close to your face. Why? A friend of mine who's an ophthalmologist says it's likely because eyelash hairs are spaced similarly to pubic hairs. Again, an eye doctor (an optometrist or an ophthalmologist) is a good place to start for any suspected pubic lice on your eyelashes. Finally, if you experience ongoing redness, irritation, or eye discharge, or if you have questions about your eye health, check in with a health care provider ASAP so as to avoid further problems or damage to your eyesight. There is no need to feel embarrassed: truly, this happens more often than many people would like to admit. Next time, don't let your partner come on your face or, if you do, use a hand shield maneuver to protect your eyes from his ejaculation. Your eyes will thank you.

27. What to do if . . . he experiences excessive pre-ejaculation—enough to wet through his clothes

This isn't likely to be a health problem. However, if a man feels embarrassed about wetting his pants this way, he can check in with a health care provider. There have been several case reports of men being successfully treated with medication for this issue.[16] Other men just wear two pairs of underwear on dates, so they don't have to worry about soaking through their clothes when they lean in for a kiss. Just as some women get extremely wet when they feel aroused, so do some men. Remember: we all have our own individual body quirks. The more we can accept each other's quirks and peculiarities, the better sex can be.

Sex Smarts Quiz

1. If a man's penis makes a popping or snapping sound during sex, it's a good idea to
    a. Get him to the emergency room
    b. Do nothing—maybe it will get better on its own
    c. Continue with sex
2. True or false: Uncircumcised men cannot wear condoms.
3. A masturbation sleeve with a hole at either end may be a particularly helpful sex toy for sex with a man whose penis is
    a. On the small side
    b. On the large side
    c. Circumcised
    d. Uncircumcised

Answers
    1. a
    2. false
    3. b

Chapter 3
The Paper Gown and You: Sexual Health Matters

S ome of the most common sex questions I receive at the Kinsey Institute and through my columns, blog, and classroom teaching are about sexual health.

Students and strangers aren't the only ones who ask me questions about sexual health though. My friends and family also have a great deal of curiosity. Recently, on a beautiful late summer evening, I joined a group of five or six girlfriends at a friend's house. We were sitting in her living room, drinking wine and talking—and often laughing—about our lives, relationships, exes, and work, the way we women often do. At some point, we started talking about various health issues and the conversation wound its way to the nitty-gritty details of gynecological exams. There was a lot of uncertainty among this group of friends (a group of women in their late twenties to early forties) about Pap tests, pelvic exams, vaginal pain, itching, HPV vaccines, and what should be a part of a normal GYN exam. In my experience, most women—no matter how smart, well-educated, or inquisitive—haven't been told much about gynecological health issues by their moms, teachers, or health care providers. We're all a bit in the dark. Many of us aren't quite sure what it is our doctors are doing when they're "down there." And some issues never stop being important. For example, even if you are in an exclusive, monogamous relationship and you and your partner don't have sex with anyone else, it's a good idea to stay up to date on information about sexually transmissible infections (STIs) so you can teach your daughters, sons, nieces, or nephews about them or so you can share the information with a friend. And given how many preteens and teenagers are more comfortable asking sex questions of adults who aren't their parents, if you're a school teacher, counselor, or aunt, you can never know too much about sexual health.

This chapter is meant to provide you with a solid update on sexual health issues that are important to many women. Some issues are familiar to many of us (like vaginal itching or burning) whereas others are less common but still important for women to learn about so they can be prepared if the issue happens to them, a friend, or a child (such as having vulvar problems from bike riding).

GREAT (GYN) EXPECTATIONS

Even women who regularly go to the gynecologist aren't always sure what their health care provider is accomplishing through a routine GYN exam. A number of my friends and students say that they generally stare at the ceiling or make small talk with their gynecologist while being examined. My doctor talks to me about triathlons (we both run, swim, and bike, though I suspect he takes it more seriously than I do) and he asks me about my work. Or I ask him GYN-related questions my students have asked me that I've been unable to answer on my own. We also, of course, talk about my body and my health—after all, that's why I'm there! Everyone has their own way of going through a GYN exam.

And although some health care providers make great efforts to involve women in the exam and use a mirror to point out their vulvar parts (and maybe even let them see inside to view their cervix), many of them are content to do the exam quietly and then move on to the next patient. This is too bad because it means that women aren't always sure what kinds of tests they are getting—or potentially what kinds of tests their health care provider has chosen, for whatever reason, not to conduct. My advice? Talk to this person. Ask questions such as "What are you doing?" or "What kinds of things are you looking for?" And if you have questions about your health, write them down on the intake form, let the nurse know, or let your health care provider know early in the visit (preferably before the pelvic exam begins) rather than wait until they're about to walk out the door. The more time they have to answer your questions, the better your visit is likely to be.

Most of the time, you can expect a few basic things to happen at an annual GYN exam (also sometimes called one's "annual exam"):

• **Paperwork.** There's no escaping it: nearly all clinics and doctor's offices ask you to complete a range of paperwork that involves questions about your own health as well as your family health history. If you don't know much about your family health history, ask your parents, siblings, grandparents, or others who might be able to help you fill in the blanks. If you have questions about your health or special concerns you want to talk about (such as painful sex, vaginal itching, a lump in your breast, unprotected sex you recently had, pregnancy, or fertility), write your question on the intake questionnaire.

• **A general exam.** Once you're called from the waiting room, the more formal intake begins. This general part of the exam is often done by a nurse and may involve taking your height, weight, and blood pressure (normally, your clothes are still on). The nurse might also ask when your last period was, so try to come into the office knowing this information. Again, if you have questions or concerns that you want to make sure to talk about with your health care provider, it's a good idea to let the nurse know (though she or he might ask you about it after they read your intake questionnaire comments). This is also a good time to state whether you would like a nurse to be present in the room during your gynecological exam. The nurse might also ask you to pee in a cup so that they can conduct urine testing.

• **Changing into a gown.** After intake, you might be sent back to the waiting room or you might be taken directly back to the exam room (offices vary in how they manage this part). Once you're in an exam room, the nurse will likely ask you to change into a paper or cloth "gown" and then typically leave the room so you can have privacy to change. It's a good idea to take off all your clothes and then change into your gown, including your bra, as health care providers often do a clinical breast exam (meaning that they feel your breasts and areas around your underarms) to check for abnormalities such as lumps.

• **Small talk.** Once your health care provider (e.g., your gynecologist, nurse practitioner, or physician's assistant) enters the room, they will often introduce themselves if it's your first visit. Even if you've been going to the same provider for years, this is the "small talk" phase where they ask how you're doing. This is the perfect time to ask the questions that are on your mind. Write your questions down on a piece of paper in advance and bring them with you if you're worried you will forget—I always do this for my annual exams and it's been very helpful. By asking questions before the pelvic exam starts, you clue your provider in to what they should be looking for. As an example, if you've been having painful sex or vaginal itching, they can make certain to look more carefully for unusual causes of pain or itching that they might otherwise not look for as closely.

• **Clinical breast exam.** As I mentioned earlier, many health care providers examine women's breasts as part of an annual exam. This may occur before or after the pelvic exam. Your provider might also ask you to breathe in and out while they use a stethoscope to listen to your heart and lungs.

• **External genital exam.** At some point, your health care provider will probably ask you to scoot your hips/butt to the edge of the exam table. This is when what women normally think of as the "GYN exam" actually begins. You may not even notice it, but health care providers typically start by looking at a woman's vulva and perianal area (the area around the anus) to make sure that all is well. With a relatively quick look, they can check for any discoloration, lumps, bumps, discharge, or areas of inflammation that may be signs of benign (noncancerous) or cancerous conditions. If they notice a red inflamed area, they might ask if you're experiencing any pain. If they notice a white patch of skin, they might ask if you've had any genital itching and may recommend taking a quick biopsy (which is a sample of your tissue) to be sent to the lab. Asking for a biopsy doesn't necessarily mean that your provider is worried about cancer; rather, white patches of genital skin are sometimes a sign of a noncancerous skin condition called lichen sclerosus. A biopsy is an important way to get a more accurate diagnosis.

• **Pelvic exam.** After the vulva (external genital) exam, the health care provider will use a speculum to look at the vagina and cervix. Smaller-sized speculums are available, so let your provider know if you have a history of painful GYN exams, painful sex, or difficulties with tampon use. A **Pap test** is often, but not always, conducted during a woman's pelvic exam. It is used to look at the health of your cervix and to test for abnormal changes. It does not test for STIs, so if it has been a while since you've been tested for STIs, including HIV, or if you have had unprotected oral, vaginal, or anal sex since your last STI test, let your health care provider know. Providers will also generally check internal organs using their glove-covered fingers and/or hand.

• **The news.** Many health care providers are sensitive to the fact that being naked and covered only in a paper or cloth gown with one's legs spread open can be a vulnerable position to be in. Many women find it an uncomfortable, or at least awkward, experience. For this reason, after the exam is over many providers will leave the room and ask the woman to get dressed, then meet with you in their office. Sometimes the health care provider simply returns to the exam room to talk. By regrouping after the exam, fully clothed, some women feel more comfortable talking about their health issues with their provider and asking any additional questions.

Some health care providers also conduct what's called a **rectovaginal exam** as part of the pelvic exam. This involves their briefly inserting a lubricated, glove-covered finger into your anus and rectum at the same time that a lubricated, glove-covered finger is inserted into your vagina. This brief exam is done to check for any masses that might signal problems such as large cysts or even early signs of uterine or ovarian cancers. Although my gynecologist does this annually, about half my friends say their doctor has never done this. I'm not sure why this is: rectovaginal exams are a widely recommended practice, don't typically hurt or cause discomfort (their gloved finger should be very well lubricated), and are actually quite quick to perform. And, at least as far as I'm concerned, the potential benefits of my doctor finding out something important about my health far outweigh any momentary awkwardness I experience from having his finger in my butt. (There's really no delicate way to put that, is there?)

THE TESTS YOU DON'T WANT TO MISS

Most of us take risks when we have sex—at least some of the time. I've certainly walked away from sexual encounters wondering if I stopped using condoms too soon with my boyfriend at the time. Even those who are good about using condoms don't always take every possible step to protect themselves. Sometimes people start having sex without a condom on and then put it on halfway through sex (not the best idea).[1] And how often have you truly worn latex gloves for fingering or hand jobs? Then there's the issue of using condoms for fellatio (blow jobs) and dental dams for cunnilingus (oral sex performed on women): although most of us know that STIs can be passed through oral sex, condoms and dams are rarely used during oral sex.[2] The truth about sex is that people often touch, lick, kiss, and suck on each other's body parts, skin to skin and tongue to skin. We get naked and, for better or worse and often in spite of knowing better, we take risks with one another. Sometimes these risks feel "worth it" and other times we regret them. For these reasons, we should all be better informed about STIs, testing, and treatment.

STI testing is included in some, but not all, GYN exams. In the US, the American College of Obstetricians and Gynecologists (ACOG) and the US Centers for Disease Control and Prevention (CDC) recommend that sexually active women age twenty-five and younger receive routine testing for chlamydia and gonorrhea. This is because a large number of women in this age group have these two common bacterial STIs and, if left untreated, either one can cause a range of reproductive health problems, including problems with fertility. However, not all health care providers follow these recommendations, and in 2007 ACOG issued a statement about this problem, noting that more than half of women who should be getting routinely screened are not. This means that there are an enormous number of women who are at risk of STIs such as chlamydia and don't even know it, and there are also many women over age twenty-five who are also at risk and who aren't regularly tested for STIs. My professional advice is to:

• **Tell your health care provider about your sexual behavior,** including whether or not you have oral sex, vaginal sex, and anal sex as well as how often you use condoms (if at all) and the number of sex partners you have had. If your health care provider doesn't ask you about your sex life, try opening the conversation by saying something like, "I have some questions about my sexual health. Can we talk about that for a few minutes?"

• **Ask if you are being tested for STIs and, if so, which ones you are being tested for.** Although young women are often tested for chlamydia and gonorrhea, that's usually it—and again, many don't get STI testing at all even though they should be. When STI testing does occur, health care providers typically don't test for everything (even though many women mistakenly believe that if they are having a GYN exam, they're getting a thorough STI test). If you want to know if you have HPV, herpes, chlamydia, gonorrhea, syphilis, HIV/AIDS, or any other STI, you need to ask your health care provider about STI testing.

Remember: this is your health so ask anything you want to. Gynecologists often take care of many aspects of women's health, so it's okay (and encouraged) to ask about health issues such as cholesterol, diabetes, thyroid function, feeling tired or stressed, feeling sad or depressed, or wondering if you have a cold or the flu. In fact, many insurance plans will allow women to identify their gynecologist as their primary care physician. Rather than seeing two different providers each year for primary care and gyn exams, it can be convenient to only see one. If you've decided you want your gynecologist to serve as your primary care physician, let them know this; that way, they can be sure to do all the other kinds of health care exams (like occasional blood work) instead of just paying attention to your "down-there care." Think of it as one-stop shopping for your health.

Be on the Lookout

Ovarian cancer is difficult to detect in its early stages and unfortunately all too many women are diagnosed too late for effective, lifesaving treatment. However, when found at an early stage, ovarian cancer has a very high five-year survival rate (above 90 percent). Be on the lookout for early warning signs of ovarian cancer, which may include bloating, back pain, painful sex, abdominal swelling, appetite loss, unexplained weight gain or loss, vaginal bleeding, frequent urination or incontinence, constipation, fatigue, indigestion, or an enlarged clitoris. Although many women experience some or many of these symptoms on occasion (meaning that they "come and go" or don't last very long), let your health care provider know if you experience them often or on an ongoing basis. Learn more from the American Cancer Society (www.cancer.org), the American College of Obstetricians and Gynecologists' patient section of their website (www.acog.org), or the National Ovarian Cancer Coalition (www.ovarian.org).

TEN THINGS EVERY WOMAN SHOULD KNOW ABOUT SEXUALLY TRANSMISSIBLE INFECTIONS

1. There are more than a hundred strains of the human papillomavirus (HPV). Some of these are called "high-risk" strains, as they are linked to cancers of the cervix and vulva (in women), the penis (in men), and the anus, head, and neck (in both women and men). Others are called "low risk" strains and are more often linked to noncancerous health issues such as genital warts, which can come and go. Genital warts are sometimes more likely to reemerge when a person's immune system is stressed. Smokers may be more likely to have wart reoccurrences. Trauma to the skin, such as shaving, can provoke warts to return too—one young woman I know found that her genital warts would return when she shaved her bikini area.

2. HPV is the most common STI in the US. A 2007 study in the *Journal of the American Medical Association* found that 26.8 percent of women in the US ages fourteen to fifty-nine had HPV (prevalence was highest—44.8 percent—among women ages twenty to twenty-four).[3] HPV can be transmitted during vaginal sex, anal sex, and (it seems, based on some studies) likely during oral sex too. Using male or female condoms during sex can reduce the risk of transmission. There is no known cure for HPV, and the course of HPV is not entirely clear. What we know is this: most sexually active people are exposed to HPV infection; however, it doesn't cause problems for most people. The problems that it sometimes causes (e.g., cervical changes that result in abnormal Pap test results and genital warts) often improve on their own; however, HPV infection can lie dormant for months or years without causing noticeable symptoms. Therefore, just because a person has never noticed a genital wart or had an abnormal Pap test, this doesn't mean they don't have HPV.

3. Chlamydia is the most common bacterial STI in the US and is particularly prevalent among women ages fifteen to twenty-four. Chlamydia can be passed during oral, vaginal, or anal sex. Again, condom use can greatly reduce the risk of transmission because it blocks fluid sharing between partners. The good news is that chlamydia can be cured with certain antibiotics prescribed by a health care provider. This is one of the most important STIs to get tested for because, if left untreated, it can result in fertility problems for women and men.

4. The herpes simplex virus—commonly known as "herpes"—can affect the genitals or a person's mouth. When the herpes simplex virus (HSV) shows up on the genitals, it's called "genital herpes" and when it shows up on the mouth, it's called "oral herpes" (or you might have heard people call them "cold sores" or "fever blisters"). Herpes can be transmitted during oral sex, vaginal sex, and anal sex, though condoms can reduce the risk of transmission when used from the start to the end of sex. According to the CDC, about one in six Americans ages fourteen to forty-nine has genital herpes.[4] Although some people think that herpes can only be passed during an outbreak, it can actually be passed even when no sores or lesions are present. That means that even though your partner's genitals "look good" they are not necessarily STI-free.

5. There is no known cure for herpes; however, some prescription antiviral medications can greatly reduce how often and how severe a person's herpes outbreaks are. Antiviral medications can also reduce the risk of passing it to a sexual partner, so couples in which one person has herpes and the other does not should talk to their health care providers about this possibility. People who get herpes often notice symptoms (such as painful sores or lesions on or around their genitals) within two weeks of transmission. But again, not everyone will notice symptoms. I know one woman who didn't have her first genital herpes outbreak until fifteen years after transmission. She knew it had been fifteen years because she hadn't had sex with anyone in the fifteen years since her divorce from her husband, who she later learned had genital herpes.

6. You can't judge a book, or someone's genitals, by its "cover." Many people mistakenly think that if their partner's genitals "look fine," there is no STI risk. This isn't true: For example, herpes isn't only contagious during an outbreak. A person can get herpes from their partner even if their partner doesn't have any visible sores or lesions. The same is true of genital warts, and many genital warts are so small they can't be seen well with the naked eye, or else they look like little pimples. Also, most people with chlamydia don't have any noticeable symptoms, which is why STI testing is so important.

7. Syphilis is sneaky. It's sneaky in the sense that, because it's a bacterial STI, many people think that it's easily protected against by using condoms. And while it's true that condom use can greatly reduce the risk of getting or passing syphilis, there are exceptions. In cases where someone has a sore or lesion from syphilis, if the condom doesn't cover the sore/lesion, syphilis may be passed even with good condom use. Syphilis can be passed during oral, vaginal, or anal sex and can cause death if left untreated (which is rare in the US and UK). On the bright side, it can be easily cured when caught in an early stage.

8. Gonorrhea is becoming more difficult to cure. It used to be that gonorrhea was very easy to cure. While it still is in most cases, certain strains of gonorrhea have developed that are resistant to antibiotics typically used to get rid of the infection.[5-6] If you test positive for gonorrhea, follow your health care provider's recommendations regarding treatment, and follow up to make sure that the infection goes away. Like most STIs, gonorrhea can be passed through oral, vaginal, or anal sex. Condom use can greatly reduce the risk of transmission.

9. HIV/AIDS doesn't only happen to gay men. Although men who have sex with men make up a disproportionately large share of HIV infections, they're not the only ones infected with HIV/AIDS. Myths that suggest HIV/AIDS is a "gay disease" hurt everyone: they further stigmatize gay men and they also put at risk other people who perhaps don't take the precautions they should to protect themselves and their partners. Talk to your health care provider about HIV. Get tested for HIV and make sure your present and future partners get tested too. Know that condom use can enormously reduce the risk of HIV transmission, so use a condom from start to finish when you have sex. HIV is most easily transmitted through anal sex or vaginal sex but can also, more rarely, be passed through oral sex.

10. Having an STI doesn't have to ruin your sex life. Most women and men will have an STI, or have a partner with an STI, at some point in their lives—even if they don't know it. STIs only have as much stigma attached to them as we allow. If we would all start talking openly about getting tested for STIs and asking partners to get tested for STIs, including HIV, it would go a long way toward normalizing safer sex and making everyone feel more accepted and reassured about their STI status. Some STIs can be cured. Even those we don't yet have cures for (such as herpes, HPV, and HIV) can be treated or managed in ways that make people's lives, including their sex lives, easier. In short, having an STI can change some aspects of your life—prompting you to talk to sexual partners about your STI status or to begin using condoms every time you have sex—but you can still have a happy, meaningful, fun, experimental, and sexy sex life.

You Can Never Know Too Much

Learning about STIs and HIV can save your life, your partner's life, or that of your children or students. On the Centers for Disease Control and Prevention's website (cdc.gov) you can read through and print easy-to-read fact sheets about each of the major STIs. And if you're raising teenagers or young adults, or teaching/mentoring teenagers, check out Get Yourself Tested (gytnow.org), a collaboration between CDC and MTV that has been effective in getting more teenagers and young adults to get STI testing.

THE MOST IMPORTANT SEX TECHNIQUE ADULTS CAN LEARN FROM TEENAGERS

Findings from my research team's National Survey of Sexual Health and Behavior were clear: teenagers were overwhelmingly good at using condoms.[7] Most sexually active adolescent men and women reported using a condom with their most recent partner, whether that person was a relationship partner or a casual partner. But adults? The data were less encouraging. Take a look, for example, at the low numbers of adult women and men who reported using a condom during their most recent sexual event with a casual partner:

- Among those ages eighteen to twenty-four, only 47 percent of men and 31 percent of women used a condom with a casual partner.
- For those ages twenty-five to twenty-nine with casual partners, 53 percent of men and 42 percent of women used a condom.
- Fifty-eight percent of men and 31 percent of women in their thirties used a condom with their casual partner.
- Among those in their forties, 36 percent of men and 20 percent of men used a condom with their casual partner.
- Twenty-eight percent of men and 24 percent of women in their fifties used a condom with their casual partner.
- For those in their sixties with casual partners, 18 percent of men and 32 percent of women used a condom.
- Among those ages seventy or greater, only 7 percent of men and none of the women in our study reported using a condom with their most recent casual partner.

The bottom line is that we adults can learn some things about sex from teenagers. Whatever your age, it's important to become comfortable buying condoms, keeping them on hand, and carrying them with you when you go out if there's even a slight chance you'll wind up having oral, vaginal, or anal sex with someone you don't know or whose STI history is anyone's guess. Of course, condoms aren't only for those who are hooking up or dating; even some long-partnered or married couples use condoms when they have sex. After all, condoms are highly effective methods of birth control.

Then there's the issue of condoms and oral sex. There is increasing evidence that HPV, possibly transmitted through oral sex, is linked to head and neck cancers[8-9]—something that has made major news headlines in recent years (HPV, sometimes transmitted through anal sex, is also linked to anal cancer). For many people, these headlines have served as a reminder that STIs can be transmitted through oral sex. Chlamydia, gonorrhea, herpes, HPV, syphilis, and, rarely, HIV can all be transmitted through oral sex whether your partner is a man or a woman. The best protection is to use a male condom during fellatio (oral sex performed on a man) or a dental dam during cunnilingus (oral sex performed on a woman). If you're turned off by the way condoms taste, choose an unlubricated condom or dental dam and put flavored lubricant on it. Not only is it tastier but if you add lubricant to both sides of the condom or dam, it can make oral sex feel more slippery and more pleasurable for your partner.

— Making It Easy —

28. What to do if . . . your genitals feel numb or tingly after a bike ride

For all its many benefits (bike riding can be fun, it's an environmentally friendly "green" form of transportation, and it can be great exercise), bike riding can also cause some uncomfortable or unusual symptoms in women and men. For example, some women experience numbness or tingling sensations on their vulva in association with bike riding. Some women notice these sensations during or immediately following a bike ride. Other women notice these genital symptoms only sporadically but during times when they are riding more often, or for longer periods of time, than usual. There have also been documented instances of women having one of their labia majora swell up to be noticeably larger than the other, something that has also been linked with bike riding.[10] Some research shows that men who are avid cyclists have a higher risk of erectile difficulties.[11]

Fortunately, none of this means that people should necessarily give up bike riding. Rather, if you have genital sensations related to numbness, tingling, or swelling that you feel may be related to your bike riding, mention this to your health care provider. It is possible that he or she may refer you to a neurologist: a doctor who specializes in issues related to nerves. Alternatively, your health care provider may simply suggest some changes to your bike riding. He or she might suggest wearing padded bicycle shorts, changing your bike saddle (the seat) to a more genital-friendly version, or occasionally rising up from the saddle during flat, easy parts of the bike ride to give your genitals a break. After all, sitting on a bike seat for long periods of time can put pressure on the genitals. To the extent that you can ease this pressure, it will be better for your genitals.

What Do Neurologists Have to Do with Sex?

Women bike riders who have numb, tingly genitals aren't the only ones who may benefit from talking to a neurologist about their sexual health. If you or your partner develop headaches during sex or at the point of orgasm, or if you or your partner temporarily black out after sex, ask your health care provider whether you should see a neurologist. There are many benign reasons for sex-related headaches or blacking out, but if the symptoms get worse or more frequent, or if you simply have questions about them, it's always a good idea to mention them to your health care provider and/or see a neurologist.

29. What to do if . . . you get an abnormal Pap test result

First, don't panic. Many women get abnormal Pap test results. The (amazingly) good news is that the vast majority of women—about 85 percent—who have abnormal Pap test results go back to having normal ones within a year. Chances are, you will be one of them.

Second, do follow your health care provider's recommendations for follow-up care. Based on certain elements of the Pap test results as well as your own personal health history, your health care provider may ask you to return in three or six months for a follow-up Pap test. Another option is that they might ask you to return sooner than that for a colposcopy, a test that involves looking more closely at your cervix and possibly taking small biopsies from your cervix to check more specifically on its health and to make sure you don't have cancer.

If you're scheduled for a colposcopy, ask your nurse or doctor what you can do to help minimize discomfort during the procedure. Some health care providers will recommend that their patients take something for pain (such as ibuprofen) or relaxation before the exam. Other health care providers do not. The procedure is not necessarily painful. However, women are all different. Just as some women find it painful to get a shot or to have their blood drawn, some women find a colposcopy more uncomfortable than other women do. If you are sensitive to pain or anxiety during medical exams or medical care, let your health care provider know. And remember: one of the best things you can do for your sexual and reproductive health is to have a GYN exam once each year or as recommended by your health care provider, and to have Pap tests and follow-up care as recommended by your health care provider.

Third, try to remember that getting an abnormal Pap test is common. Many women can relate, including perhaps several of your friends, coworkers, or family members. Some women feel ashamed to learn that they have an abnormal Pap test result, particularly as many abnormal Pap test results are linked to HPV infection, which is linked to sex. I would love for us to get to a place in society in which sex isn't linked to shame. Having had sex—even lots of sex, or with a number of partners—doesn't make you a bad person. Going to see a health care provider and getting a Pap test, at least in my opinion, makes you a very responsible, smart person. Good for you for taking care of your health.

30. What to do if . . . you have excessive or colored vaginal discharge

Easy: let your health care provider know about any new, excessive, or unusually colored discharge that you notice. And if no one has ever mentioned this before, allow me: in addition to checking out your vulva at least once a month to understand what looks and feels normal for you, I would also encourage you to become familiar with your underwear. Yes, your underwear! Here's why: you've probably noticed over the years that vaginal discharge appears on your underwear. Vaginal discharge, of course, is completely normal and a fancy way that the vagina has to clean itself out on an ongoing basis. Wearing white or light-colored underwear can help you become familiar with the shades of your normal vaginal secretions, which will typically be clear, light yellow, or white depending on the phase of your menstrual cycle. If you notice a change to the color or thickness of this discharge, let your health care provider know. If you've had unprotected sex, or if you have other symptoms (such as itching, burning, genital pain, bladder pain, or back pain), share that information with your doctor or nurse as well.

There are also some things you can do at home to try to get rid of the discharge. Steer clear of feminine hygiene products such as douches, powders, sprays, and genital deodorants, as these can irritate women's genitals and contribute to vaginal discharge. If you've recently started using a new lubricant or a new bath wash, soap, or laundry detergent, try going without that product for several days or a week to see if the discharge clears up. In some instances, vaginal discharge changes in response to an irritating product and stopping use of that product can help the discharge go away.

31. What to do if . . . you're diagnosed with chlamydia

Most women who have chlamydia will have no noticeable symptoms at all. Those who do may notice abnormal vaginal discharge or a burning sensation while peeing. If left untreated, the infection can spread into the uterus and fallopian tubes, and symptoms may include painful intercourse, bleeding in between menstrual periods, or lower back pain.

If you receive a chlamydia diagnosis, follow your health care provider's recommendation for treatment. Chlamydia can be cured by taking certain antibiotics available by prescription. Notify your sexual partner(s) so that they can be tested and treated too. Depending on where you live and the policies of certain medical clinics, your health care provider may even send you home with a prescription for your sexual partner(s). This is because chlamydia is very easily transmitted during sex, so if you have had unprotected sex with a partner, it is very likely that you have given it to him or her (or that your most recent partner gave it to you, depending on the situation). It is also possible that you have had the infection for a long time and given it to more than one person, or that they have had the infection for a long time and not only given it to you, but to multiple partners. In any case, if you have chlamydia, you can at least count on the fact that there's some-one who gave it to you who may be in need of treatment (which is why some health care providers send home a prescription for one's partner).

Even though chlamydia can be cured with certain antibiotics, it is not an instant cure. It is often recommended that patients continue to use con-doms when they have sex for at least two weeks after they begin treatment, and then that they return to a clinic to be tested again for chlamydia to make sure that it has been successfully treated before returning to con-domless sex. Ask your health care provider what he or she recommends for you in terms of condom use and follow-up testing.

If you don't wish to tell your present or past partners that you have chlamydia, but you still want to do the world a favor, ask your health care provider whether they have a "partner notification" program. This involves giving your health care provider the name and contact information (phone or email) of present and/or past partners who may have given you chlamy-dia, or who may have gotten it from you. Rather than you having to notify them, your health care provider calls and says something along the lines of "You have been listed as a sexual contact of someone who has been diag-nosed with chlamydia" and then provides information to that person about testing and treatment options. They don't share your name; rather, the goal is to get more people tested and treated so that the STI stops being spread to others. If you have questions about the confidential nature of your health care provider's partner notification program, ask them.

Remember, too, that chlamydia is the most common bacterial STI in many countries. You didn't do anything wrong or bad to get chlamydia, and you deserve to feel proud of yourself for taking good enough care of your health that you got tested for it. Going forward, remember that condom use and regular STI testing (for you and your partner) can help prevent further infections.

32. What to do if . . . someone you want to climb into bed with has genital warts

This can be a challenging issue for many people. If you feel only so-so about the person or feel only mildly sexually or romantically interested in them, then you might feel it's not worth the risk to have sex with them and possibly wind up with genital warts. You might decide that, as nice or as attractive as they seem, you would rather not gamble with getting the infetion. Of course, if you have genital warts yourself, there is little risk in that sense, but you should still consider using condoms to prevent passing other STIs.

HPV Vaccines

There are currently two types of HPV vaccines available in the US and many other countries: Gardasil, which helps to prevent four strains of HPV (two linked to cancers and two linked to genital warts), and Cervarix, which protects against two strains of HPV linked to cancers. In addition to cervical cancer, these high-risk strains of HPV have also been linked to cancers of the vagina, vulva, and anus. Both vaccines are approved for use among girls and young women. At this writing, only Gardasil is approved for use in boys and young men. Although HPV vaccines will be most effective among individuals who have not yet had sex (and thus not yet been exposed to HPV), it can still be given to women and men who have previously had sex. That said, if you have already been infected with all of the HPV strains the vaccine covers, there's unlikely to be any benefit in you receiving the vaccine—ask your healthcare provider if the vaccine is a good option for you.

Although many people are in favor of HPV vaccination, some people are critical of the vaccine because they suggest that young people who don't want to get an STI shouldn't be having sex anyway. And some people have heard a great deal of misinformation about one or both HPV vaccines, making them feel suspicious. Because both HPV vaccines are relatively new to the US market, it is understandable that some people want to wait until there are more studies on the vaccines' safety before they or their children are vaccinated. Then again, many health care providers believe that the benefits of the vaccine (e.g., not getting high-risk strains of HPV) far outweigh the risks, which at this point appear to be quite low. The vast majority of women and men who are vaccinated for HPV seem to do very well with the vaccine and don't experience noticeable side effects. If you are considering vaccinating for HPV for yourself or your daughter, I would encourage you to find out more from your health care provider and to visit reputable, trustworthy web sites such as those of the Centers for Disease Control and Prevention (www.cdc.gov) and the American College of Obstetricians and Gynecologists (www.acog.org). Women who receive the HPV vaccine should still continue to get Pap tests as recommended by their health care provider, particularly as neither HPV vaccine can prevent cervical cancer or other kinds of cancers—they can only reduce the risk of them.

If you decide you'd like to have sex with this person, remember that using condoms offers some (but not complete) protection against genital warts and significant protection against HIV, chlamydia, gonorrhea, and some other STIs. Remember, too, that there need not be a "rush" to have sex. If your partner has warts and you do not, why not talk to your health care provider about the Gardasil vaccine for HPV? Two of the strains it protects against are linked to most cases of genital warts (see sidebar on HPV vaccines). If you have had the Gardasil vaccine, or if you get it before you have sex with this person, then you will have a very low risk of acquiring genital warts.

It's worth noting, too, that although genital warts aren't painful like herpes sores can be, they may be linked to some health risks. For example, women who have a skin disorder called lichen sclerosus (LS) on their genitals have a slightly increased risk of developing vulvar cancer at some point in their lives (albeit the risk remains small at about 4 or 5 percent). However, women who have genital lichen sclerosus *and* who have genital warts appear to be at an even greater risk for vulvar cancer, for reasons that are not well understood. This is not a reason to panic. After all, LS can be very well managed by thoughtful health care providers and good follow-up care and there are many things women can do to reduce their cancer risk, such as manage stress, eat a healthy diet rich in colorful vegetables, and not smoke (all steps that many of us can benefit from). It is a good reminder, though, that decisions about STI risk are important and that they're different for every woman.

33. What to do if . . . you're diagnosed with herpes

Genital herpes is very common: according to recent data from the Centers for Disease Control and Prevention, about one in five women and about one in nine men ages fourteen to forty-nine are infected with herpes simplex virus-2 on their genitals.[12] Unfortunately, many people have no idea that they have genital herpes and they may spread it to sexual partners without meaning to. If you have genital herpes, ask your health care provider about antiviral medications that may reduce how often you have outbreaks, how severe or painful your outbreaks are, and the likelihood of transmitting herpes to sexual partners. Even if you're being treated for herpes, you can still transmit it to others—the risk is just lower—so you should still tell sexual partners about your diagnosis. Keep condoms in mind too: when used correctly and consistently, they reduce the risk of transmitting herpes (even though they cannot completely protect against herpes, as condoms cannot cover all of one's genital skin). Finally, some people with herpes find it helpful to connect with local or Internet-based herpes support groups, particularly in regard to tips for talking to sexual partners about their diagnosis. Check out www.datingwithherpes.org for a variety of resources related to sex, dating, and relationships for people with herpes.

34. What to do if . . . your (supposedly) monogamous partner is diagnosed with an STI

This one is never "easy," but I do hope some of this information makes it easier to figure out what it means for you. It's important to know that one cannot get an STI such as chlamydia, gonorrhea, trichomoniasis, HIV, genital HPV, or herpes from a toilet seat or from shaking hands with another person. That said, there have been instances in which people appear to have contracted herpes from using a hookah, and if you or your partner got oral herpes that way and then performed oral sex on one another, one could conceivably get herpes on the genitals that way. That would be a rare and unlikely instance.

In most cases, however, if you think you are in a monogamous sexual relationship with your partner (meaning that both of you have agreed not to have oral, vaginal, or anal sex with other people) and you suddenly get an STI—even though you had both tested negative for STIs earlier in your relationship—then it is highly likely that your partner has had sex with someone else. Unfortunately, people sometimes lie about having sex with others. Even if you confront your partner, they may not admit to having had sex with another person. They may tell you that you're crazy or even accuse you of cheating (of course, if you are the one who had sex with another person, you should own up to your behavior and make decisions in the future that protect you and your partner from infection).

If you suspect that your partner has had sex with someone else—or if you are the one who has strayed—it is time for a discussion about your romantic and sexual relationship. What expectations do you have for one another? What makes it easy or difficult for you to stay monogamous? If you stay together, do you want to stay monogamous or do you both want to open your relationship so that one or both of you is allowed some form of sexual expression with other people? If you open up your relationship, you will also want to be clear about "rules" such as the importance of using condoms with other people (and maybe even when you have sex with each other) and getting regularly tested for STIs. You may decide, too, that you no longer want to stay together, which is another option. Whatever you decide, know that you can get through this, alone or together, and move on with life.

35. What to do if . . . you bleed during or after intercourse

Women should always let their health care provider know if they experience vaginal bleeding during or after vaginal intercourse. It may be that you have fragile skin because of low estrogen or a skin disorder and the fragile skin is giving way to tears or cuts during sex. Then again, the bleeding may be coming from inside your body. It could be due to what's called a friable cervix or to fibroids (lumps that grow on your uterus). More rarely, bleeding during sex can be a sign of ovarian cancer. Although bleeding during or after sex is often benign, it is always a symptom that deserves a thoughtful conversation with one's health care provider. And if you feel your symptoms are being ignored or not given the attention they deserve, consider getting a second opinion from another gynecologist.

Trich-y Business

Trichomoniasis (often called "trich" for short) is the most common curable STI among young women in the US yet is rarely talked about. When men get trich, they seldom show symptoms. Women, however, often experience a strong vaginal odor accompanied by a frothy, greenish-yellow vaginal discharge, discomfort or pain during sex, and possibly vaginal itching. Trich is caused by a parasite and, thankfully, can be cured with prescription medications from a health care provider. How can you prevent getting trich? You know the drill: use a condom, and ask your partner to get tested for STIs before you have sex together.

36. What to do if . . . you get a yeast infection—*again*

There are two types of women who get yeast infections: those who get them sporadically and those who have recurrent yeast infections, which are often defined as four or more yeast infections in a given year. If you get yeast infections only every now and then, chances are that you sometimes mistake vaginal itching or irritation for a yeast infection; many women think they have a yeast infection when they don't. If you are a woman who only has occasional yeast infections, count yourself lucky—and call your health care provider before you rush to the store to stock up on yeast medication or cream. Why? Because if you're wrong, you may make your symptoms worse and make it more difficult for your health care provider to eventually figure out what's causing your symptoms. Calling your nurse or doctor first gives them a chance to ask you a few basic questions about your symptoms, which increases the likelihood of a correct diagnosis, appropriate treatment, and you getting better.

If you are a woman who gets recurrent yeast infections, you're likely to be more in tune with your symptoms and may be just fine running out to the store to get the cream or medication you need. It's still a good idea to ask your health care provider their opinion on whether you should call their office each time or treat it at home on your own.

Just as there are two types of women who get yeast infections, there is also more than one type of yeast that affects women. Candida albicans is the most common culprit that overgrows and plagues women's vaginas; this kind is often treated reasonably well with over-the-counter creams or with medications. There are other kinds of yeast, however, that require different treatment options. If you have a yeast infection that is difficult to treat and that doesn't seem to improve, ask your health care provider if he or she has tested for the particular type of yeast you have (they don't always do this)— and if not, if they would be willing to. Or you might try to get a second opinion from a vulvovaginal specialist who has significant experience treating yeast infections and other vulvovaginal health issues. After all, sometimes women's vulvovaginal health issues aren't limited to yeast infections and something else may be causing you to have ongoing symptoms.

Sex Smarts Quiz

1. Which of the following reduce the risk of "catching" genital warts from an infected partner?
   a. Using a condom from start to finish during sex
   b. Having had the Gardasil vaccine prior to having sex with your partner
   c. Wishing really hard
   d. a and b only
   e. All of the above
2. A Pap test checks for
   a. Cervical changes
   b. Chlamydia
   c. Gonorrhea
   d. All of the above
3. True or False:
   All yeast infections can be easily treated using one kind of treatment.

Answers
   1. d
   2. a
   3. false

Chapter 4
Women's Orgasm: Singles, Multiples, and the One That Got Away

I f I had a dollar for every time I've been asked a question about women's orgasm, I would be a very wealthy woman. Orgasm is an experience that, if it happens at all, lasts only about twenty seconds or so on average. For such a fleeting experience, it sure occupies a lot of people's sexual concerns (and excitements too). In this chapter, get ready to learn key information about women's orgasms, including

- The so-called "orgasm gap"
- How women have orgasms
- Three major nerve pathways that are important to female orgasms
- The many ways that women experience orgasm (some of them may surprise you)
- The link between orgasm and sexual variety

Orgasm is not a critical part of sex for all women or men, but it is an important aspect for many people. In a national survey of British women and men, less than half (49 percent of men and 43 percent of women) agreed or strongly agreed with a statement that said sex without orgasm cannot really be satisfying.[1] However, orgasm—both one's own and that of one's partner—is important to most women and men. In a 2011 study of more than a thousand long-term couples in five countries[2] (the men and women were between ages forty and seventy), there were several interesting orgasm-related findings, including:

1. Men highly valued their own orgasms and their partner's orgasms. On a scale of 1 to 10 (1=not at all, 10=very), the average "importance score" for men's own orgasms was 8.45. The value they placed on their partner's orgasm averaged out to be 8.53.

2. Women valued their partner's orgasms more so than their own. Using the same scale as for the men, the value women placed on their own orgasm averaged to be 7.35 whereas the value they placed on their male partner's orgasm was 7.96.

3. The more value men placed on their partner's orgasm, the more likely they were to be happy in their relationship. Men's sexual satisfaction was also linked to the value they placed on their partner's orgasm.

Again, orgasm isn't the number-one focus of sex for every person every time they have sex. However, it is one aspect of sex that matters to many women and men. For those who want to enhance this aspect of their sexual experiences, there are facts about orgasm and sexual pleasure that can make a real and noticeable difference. Here, you'll find a number of orgasm questions answered as well as a few fun facts to share with your friends or sexual partner.

The Orgasm Myth—Exploded

We women are unique in countless ways. We differ from each other in terms of our height, weight, curviness, breast size, hair color, nose size, shoe size, skin color, labia size, and the number of freckles that dot our bodies. And that's just the outside parts. We also vary in terms of our musical abilities, whether we're better with numbers or art, and how well we can sing or dance or remember the birthdays or anniversaries of our families and friends. Some women can wrap gifts more beautifully than Martha Stewart. Some women can manage an office or a large family with almost military precision. We all have our gifts and unique characteristics that make us who we are.

Orgasm isn't much different, despite what many women's magazines and so-called "sex experts" would have you believe. There are so many myths about orgasms that I hear all the time: that G Spot orgasms are more intense than clitoral orgasms, or that any woman can have an orgasm if she can find her clitoris, or that one can learn to experience orgasm for hours and hours at a time. These myths are harmful to women, particularly when some of them make women feel inadequate if they're not orgasmic or not orgasmic "enough."

The truth is that some women experience orgasm very easily, even if they don't put any effort into trying. Other women may try for months or years and never have an orgasm, or else they may have orgasms in some situations (such as when receiving oral sex) but not others (such as intercourse). Many of us are in the middle. Like most women, I can remember a time when I didn't have orgasms. When I learned to experience orgasm, it was little by little and with different types of sexual experiences (masturbation, then hand stimulation from a partner, then oral sex, and—years later—through vaginal intercourse). This is important because it goes against the way many "sex experts" divide the world: that there are women who orgasm and women who don't. The reality is that most of us will experience orgasm at some point in our lives; it may just take a little while and require some practice and learning.

One of my favorite recent scientific studies added to our understanding of how orgasm varies from woman to woman. In this study, published in a 2011 issue of *Hormones and Behavior*, researchers from Emory University and Indiana University found that in two samples of women they studied, the distance between a woman's clitoris and her urethra was linked to her likelihood of having an orgasm during sex.[3] Scientists who study sex, including me, aren't quite sure how this might work, if it's true for other women. For example, do some women's genitals allow for greater contact between the penis and the clitoris during sex? Are some women's genitals better positioned to allow the penis to stimulate the inside parts of the clitoris? Or is this anatomical difference a sign of something else—for example, that these women are different hormonally from other women? This was a preliminary research study but an important step in our understanding of how the experience of orgasm varies for women. And it reminds me that we are all different in many ways. We don't expect our hair, eyes, or breasts to all look alike: why would our orgasms all be alike?

Finally, it's important to add that this study provides just one piece of a larger orgasm puzzle. Not all orgasms involve clitoral stimulation; a minority of women experienced orgasm from breast stimulation or mental fantasy, and some women who have experienced more extensive versions of female genital circumcision, involving removal of most or all of the clitoris, report experiencing orgasm. And of course not all women have penile-vaginal intercourse, let alone experience orgasm from it. However, this study suggests that one of the many things that may matter to women's orgasmic ease has to do with how her body happens to have been formed in the womb, or how it developed as she grew into adulthood.

Orgasm, Uncovered

While scientists still have a great deal left to discover about the female orgasm, it's not a complete mystery. We are learning more and more about it all the time and these findings can help us all have more pleasurable, and often more easily orgasmic, sex.

In our recent National Survey of Sexual Health and Behavior we found evidence for the idea that orgasm truly may become easier with age, at least to some extent. Although 61 percent of women ages eighteen to twenty-four and 58 percent of women ages twenty-five to twenty-nine said that they experienced orgasm during the most recent time they had sex with a partner (which could have been oral sex, vaginal sex, anal sex, or something else such as mutual masturbation), more women reported orgasm as they grew older.[4] A total of 65 percent of women in their thirties and 69 percent of women in their forties reported experiencing orgasm during their most recent sexual event. However, we also found a sort of bell curve with more women in their thirties and forties reporting orgasm and then fewer women reporting orgasm in their fifties and sixties (in our study, 61 percent of women in their fifties and 44 percent of women in their sixties reported having an orgasm at their most recent event). In contrast, more men (above 90 percent in men younger than sixty) reported experiencing orgasm when they most recently had sex with a partner. For men, orgasm and ejaculation become more difficult with age.

What this tells me is that scientists have been correct in their finding that, particularly for women, learning to experience orgasm takes practice. Generally speaking, men tend to find it easier to orgasm than women do. Also, more young men start masturbating at earlier ages than young women, so they have more time to practice and learn what "works" for their bodies and minds. These data also tell us something else: that although orgasm gets easier with age to some extent, it's not completely true. Over time, many women experience health problems or the loss of a partner (due to illness, death, divorce, or separation), and this can result in many profound sexual changes for women in their forties, fifties, sixties, and beyond. Therefore, age doesn't automatically make for better sex or more frequent orgasms. There are always ups and downs to any stage of life.

The Value of Letting Go

In a 2011 study published in *Hormones and Behavior,* Dutch researchers examined brain scans of men and women during sexual stimulation and orgasm.[5] Building on previous research, they found that a common feature of the brain scans during sexual stimulation and orgasm is that a number of areas of our brains deactivate, or sort of "shut off," especially on the left side of the brain (which is linked to rational thinking, information processing, and controlling feelings). In contrast, the right side of the brain (which is related more to spontaneous feelings and emotions) is somewhat activated. The scientists involved in this study speculated on the importance of "letting go" as part of sexual experiences and orgasm. It can be difficult to do so, and mindfulness exercises—breathing in and out and focusing on the scents, sights, and tastes of your sexual experiences—may be of help. Read more about mindfulness exercises as they apply to sex in my first book, *Because It Feels Good: A Woman's Guide to Sexual Pleasure and Satisfaction.*

How Women Orgasm

Recent research published in the *Journal of Sexual Medicine* in 2011 added to scientists' thinking on women's orgasm. In an interesting fMRI study (which involves taking brain scans), it was discovered that stimulation of a woman's nipples activates the same part of the brain that is activated when a woman's genitals are stimulated.[6] This may help explain how it is that some women are able to experience orgasm when their nipples are stimulated.

These researchers learned another fascinating piece of information about women's orgasm. They found that stimulation of a woman's vagina activates a different part of the brain than stimulation of a woman's clitoris does. For some women, this underscores the differences they feel between an orgasm from vaginal stimulation and an orgasm from clitoral stimulation. It's not that one orgasm "type" is universally better than the other—remember, every woman is different and has her own preferences—but it does help explain why they might feel somewhat different to women. And if it's true that vaginal intercourse often stimulates both the vagina and the clitoris (as mentioned earlier in chapter 1), then these data may add to our understanding of how some orgasms feel different or more or less intense than others. Maybe combined vaginal and clitoral stimulation feels qualitatively different than stimulation of just the vagina or just the clitoris —not necessarily better or worse, but different.

Earlier research found that there are different nerve pathways involved in women's orgasms and that this may explain why some orgasms feel different to different women (for a detailed account of this, check out *The Science of Orgasm* by Barry Komisaruk, Carlos Beyer-Flores and Beverly Whipple). The clitoris, for example, sends a lot of its sensory information through the pudendal nerve, whereas the vagina is mainly supplied by the pelvic nerve and the cervix by several nerves (including the vagus nerve). If the clitoris is the main part that's stimulated, then most of the sensory information about pleasure will be conveyed through the pudendal nerve. If more than one part is stimulated (say, the vagina, clitoris, and cervix through deep vaginal inter-course) then it might be the case that sensory information floods two or three nerve pathways, "lighting up" multiple parts of the brain.

Not only are the nerve pathways different, but women stimulate these body parts and nerve pathways in all sorts of different ways. As young children, parents and other caregivers (such as preschool teachers) have reported seeing both girls and boys stimulating themselves with their hands, stuffed animals, playground equipment (such as repeatedly sliding up and down poles), blankets, and pillows. In scientific studies that ask adults about their childhood experiences, in addition to recalling playing with stuffed animals or blankets in this manner, they also sometimes say they remember stimulating themselves by dripping water on their genitals from a bathtub faucet or by sitting on top of the washing machine while it rumbled away (essentially serving as a large vibrator that also conveniently cleans one's clothes). And as teenagers or adults, women may engage in a wide range of sexual behavior that helps them experience orgasm including breast stimulation, erotic massage, masturbation with the hands, masturbation with sex toys, vaginal sex, oral sex, anal sex, sexual fantasy, fingering, and much, much more.

ORGASMS DURING EXERCISE

One of the great joys of my job is that I hear from so many people about their sex lives, and their personal stories inspire my research. For years, I would receive letters from women about their experiences having orgasms while running, lifting weights, doing sit-ups, or engaging in some other form of exercise. When I looked to the scientific literature, I found that there had never been a study on the topic and that women's and men's magazines had written more about these experiences than scientists ever had. So of course I decided I needed to conduct a study and learn more from women themselves.

In the study I conducted at Indiana University, I asked women about their experiences with what I call "exercise-induced orgasms." In the study, women wrote about a number of experiences having orgasms, often by accident, while doing sit-ups, pull-ups, yoga, or other exercises as children, teenagers, or adults. We don't particularly understand how these exercise-induced orgasms happen. Certainly some of them seem to involve friction, such as rubbing one's genitals on a bicycle seat or shimmying up a rope in PE class. For example, one woman in our study described her experience with an exercise-induced orgasm in this way:

> *I was biking up a hill . . . and I had to really grind into the pedals. This must have caused me to rub on the seat in just the right way. I thought I was starting to cramp, but soon realized it felt great. I started to get wet and thought I should stop . . . but chose not to! I came for the very first time shortly after that! Embarrassingly my friend whom I was biking with teased me about my sweating crotch. I never admitted to what had actually happened and I have tried to replicate it ever since— with no luck!*
> —Woman, age forty-one

Other women, however, describe orgasms during exercise that don't seem to be caused by friction or their clitoris rubbing up against anything in particular. Some of these instances seem to have more to do with the use of abdominal exercises (which reflects why so many people call these types of orgasms "coregasms," as they engage the core abdominal muscles). In describing this type of orgasm, one woman wrote,

> *If I engage my lower stomach muscles—the ones below my navel—I get a sharp increase in pleasure, perhaps leading to orgasm. This is particularly true if I sit in a straddle position and reach forward. Also, if I lie on my back and stretch one of my legs up, pulling it towards me, I'll probably orgasm after a minute or two.*
> —Woman, age twenty-three

Working on this study convinced me just how different women are in their experience of orgasm. Even though women in my study experienced orgasm during exercise, they had their own individual ways of doing so.

Some women experienced them while during sit-ups, while sit-ups didn't work at all for other women, who instead were able to experience orgasm while swimming, biking, or doing yoga. Again, we are all unique and need to find what is pleasurable or orgasmic for ourselves rather than try to measure up to some pretend standard of what "everybody else is doing" (especially since that's usually wrong anyway).

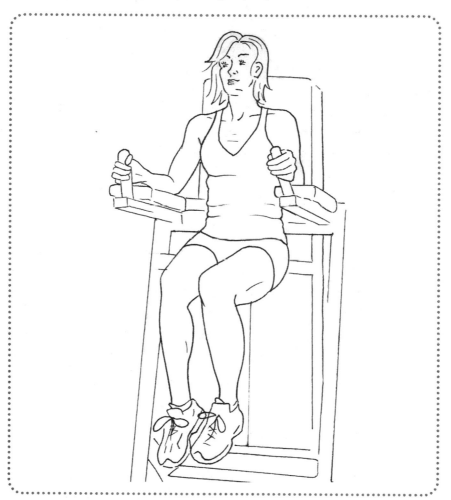

Abdominal exercises performed on the Captain's Chair (pictured) were among the most common forms of exercises that women reported led them to experience orgasm.

Four Orgasm Facts You Can Use to Entertain Your Friends

1. Breastfeeding has its surprises. While very few women experience orgasm during vaginal delivery, a larger number report experiencing feelings of sexual arousal or even orgasm while breastfeeding.[7] Because orgasms linked to breastfeeding are so rarely discussed, many women are taken aback when it happens to them and may feel ashamed, as if they have done something wrong (they haven't). This normal bodily response appears to be linked to the increase in oxytocin release that is triggered during breastfeeding. Because oxytocin is also released when women have orgasms, it can feel very similar and worry women, some of whom even quit breastfeeding their babies because of it.

2. We have ourselves an "orgasm gap." In our National Survey of Sexual Health and Behavior (NSSHB), we found that 85 percent of men (most of whom had female partners) reported that their partner had an orgasm during their most recent sex act. However, only 64 percent of women said they had an orgasm the last time they had sex.[8] We're not sure if this is because a number of women fake orgasms or because partners simply don't communicate very well about it, but the gap between the two numbers is striking, isn't it?

3. Variety is the spice of life—and orgasm. In the NSSHB, we found that greater sexual variety was linked to women's orgasm.[9] Women who reported engaging in several sex acts (for example, vaginal sex, performing oral sex, receiving oral sex) as opposed to just one or two had a greater likelihood of experiencing orgasm.

4. Orgasm can be dreamy. That is, some women—like some men—experience orgasm while they sleep. Genital arousal is linked with REM sleep, which means that several times per night blood flow increases to the genitals, resulting in greater vaginal lubrication and arousal for women and erections for men. Every now and then, an orgasm or two during sleep is an added bonus. Some women recall experiencing sex-related dreams that prompt their orgasm, but not all do.

— Making It Easy—

37. What to do if . . . you have orgasm-induced headaches

If it happens once or twice, it's probably not a big deal, though you should always mention health concerns to your doctor. If you frequently have headaches that begin when you experience orgasm, or if they're becoming more common, definitely bring this to the attention of your doctor and/or ask for a referral to a neurologist. A 2003 study of fifty-one individuals with sex-related headaches found that they were more common among men (by about three to one), but that doesn't mean women never get them.[10] Some severe headaches are linked to use of recreational drugs, such as marijuana and cocaine. Others are linked to vascular disorders, which is why such headaches should always be mentioned to one's health care provider.

38. What to do if . . . you can't have an orgasm thanks to antidepressants

Sexual side effects are common with certain antidepressants. Many people find this improves after a few weeks or a few months of taking medication. Others find that their sexual side effects don't go away, and they may become distressed by them and ask their health care provider whether it would be possible for them to switch to another antidepressant that doesn't pose as much of a risk. Sometimes this is a solution that works.

For mild depression or anxiety, some women and men find that they are able to work with a therapist to treat their problem without medication. Relaxation exercises and cognitive behavioral therapy are helpful for many people. Sometimes people see such significant improvement in their lives that they no longer need medication. For some people, however, medication is a very important part of treatment, and it may be that sexual side effects come along as an unfortunate part of the package. If you find it difficult to orgasm thanks to good old antidepressant side effects, you might try adding a vibrator to your sexual routine (whether masturbation, sex play with a partner, or intercourse). Vibration can make orgasms easier for both women and men. Others find that spending time relaxing and focusing on foreplay, amping up one's arousal, enhances the overall sexual experience and helps orgasm along. Finally, a study published in the *Journal of the American Medical Association* in 2008 found that the use of sildenafil (Viagra) may help alleviate some of the sexual side effects that are common to certain antidepressants.[11] Of course, not everyone wants to take yet another pill, but for those who are open to the idea, it is something to discuss with a health care provider.

39. What to do if . . . your orgasms aren't as strong as they used to be

As we age, so do our bodies—and, to some extent, our orgasms. Noticing a change in orgasmic feel is a normal part of aging. The muscles that surround the vagina, uterus, and anus all play a role in orgasmic contractions and, of course, muscles throughout our bodies tend to become weaker with age unless we do what we can to strengthen them. Being pregnant can also weaken women's pelvic floor muscles, which is one reason why women who have been pregnant often have a greater risk of incontinence (peeing when one doesn't mean to pee).

That said, there are several steps you can take to maintain or gain as much orgasmic strength as is possible. Kegel exercises (described in chapter 1) can help maintain or build pelvic floor muscle tone. Staying fit, particularly through cardiovascular exercise, may also help you feel more energetic, in and out of bed. As a good deal of sexual response has to do with blood flowing through one's body, it may be that cardiovascular exercises (such as walking, running, swimming, playing tennis, or basketball) will help with your experience of sexual arousal and even orgasm. Some women find that adding a vibrator to their private or partnered sex play adds more intensity to their orgasms. You might experiment with various intensities of vibration in order to see what works for you; for example, some women prefer using low-intensity vibrations to create a slow buildup that ultimately results in a more intense experience of orgasm for them. Other women find that more intense vibration is more pleasurable for them and results in a stronger orgasm. Fantasizing about sex can also help to make orgasm feel easy to come by or stronger when it occurs.

In addition, feelings of intimacy and connection cannot be overlooked in the experience of orgasm. Some women find that kissing their partner more often throughout sex helps them feel sexy, loved, lustful, or more excited—all of which can translate into a more satisfying response to sex or experience of orgasm. And for many couples, emotional intimacy begins far before they ever take off their clothes or get into bed. For many people, and especially for women, feeling as if one's partner "sees them" or "gets them" is important for sexual desire, satisfaction, and ease of orgasm.

Sex Post-cancer

Cancer and cancer treatments can impact a woman's experience of sexuality, including orgasm, and there is limited research on addressing sexual concerns following cancer treatment. Women cancer survivors who experience orgasm difficulties may require more intense stimulation in order to experience sexual pleasure or orgasm. In these cases, a multispeed vibrator (such as a Silver Bullet vibrator) or a high-intensity vibrator (such as the Hitachi Magic Wand or Accuvibe) may be good options to consider. Many women experience vaginal dryness and/or genital pain following treatment for cancer as well, and this discomfort can get in the way of a woman's ability to let go, relax, and open herself to pleasure and/or orgasm. Using a store-bought lubricant during sex can be helpful, as can using a vaginal moisturizer as directed by one's health care provider. Not all vaginal moisturizers contain estrogens, so don't let that stop you from learning more from your doctor or nurse. A number of women find that alternative therapies such as mindfulness techniques and yoga help enhance their sex lives as well. Some sex shops now make unscented and unflavored versions of sexual enhancement products (such as lubricants and body powders) to be more sensitive to the needs of cancer patients, particularly those going through chemotherapy, which can affect individuals' sense of smell and taste and vulnerability to feeling nauseous. Learn more about sexuality after cancer in *Sexy Ever After: Intimacy Post Cancer* by Patty Brisben and Keri Peterson MD and *Living Well Beyond Breast Cancer* by Marisa Weiss MD and Ellen Weiss.

40. What to do if . . . your go-to pre-baby sex position no longer results in orgasm

If orgasm is important to you, then try, try, and try some more. For reasons that are not well understood (there is strikingly little research on sex after having a baby), women's bodies and sexual response may be very different after they've given birth—sometimes in surprisingly good ways. Because these changes are not predictable, it's not as easy as suggesting that new mothers try missionary or woman on top because pleasurable and orgasmic sex may come with any number of sex positions or sex acts.

My best advice for new moms, then, is to keep an open mind and explore their sexuality as if they were starting over with a new slate. Even if missionary didn't do much for you before, it might now. Who knows? Try missionary, woman on top, reverse cowgirl, spooning, scissors, oral sex, breast play, sensuous massage, and so on. Get a book focused on sex positions and go through them, trying each at least two or three times (unless it's uncomfortable, painful, or simply doesn't appeal to you and your partner—then feel free to skip it). Try to be patient too. I know that's much easier said than done, but it can often take six or more months after having a baby to feel like oneself again sexually. Some women take longer than others, particularly if childbirth was traumatic or involved a great deal of tearing.

There is reason to be hopeful, though: just because one position doesn't feel like it used to doesn't mean that another one might not feel better than before. I hear this so often from new mothers that I believe it's worth sharing with you to encourage you in your exploration.

41. What to do if . . . you've been told that you need a hysterectomy and wonder how this will change your orgasms

Fortunately, having a hysterectomy doesn't mean doom for your orgasms. Some research has found that one of the best predictors of a woman's sex life after a hysterectomy is the sex life she had before she had the hysterectomy. In other words, if your sex life wasn't all that satisfying beforehand, a hysterectomy is unlikely to make it better (though of course other health issues may be much improved post-hysterectomy). And if you generally had a good sex life beforehand, chances are that once you recover from the procedure you should be ready to resume your sex life as before.

In a 2004 study published in the *Journal of Obstetrics and Gynecology*, researchers from Northwestern University's Feinberg School of Medicine tracked women before and after hysterectomy.[12] They found that most women didn't expect their sexual desire or orgasm to change and they were right: neither changed. What did change, however, was that they (fortunately) were less likely to experience painful sex after their hysterectomy.

This isn't to say that nothing ever changes with a hysterectomy. Sex (and your orgasms) may feel slightly different after the operation. Some women who are very tuned in to feeling their uterus contract in relation to orgasm notice the absence of those contractions after their uterus is removed. This happened to a friend of mine, who said that her orgasms initially felt less intense after her hysterectomy but, with time, she no longer noticed the absence of those contractions. She developed a "new normal" for herself. And besides, the uterus is only one part. There are still plenty of other contractions that can be felt as part of orgasm.

Some women, in addition to having part or all of the uterus removed during the hysterectomy, also have one or both ovaries removed at the same time (a procedure called an "oophorectomy"). If you are having a hysterectomy, ask your health care provider if he or she is also planning to remove your ovaries and, if so, (a) if it is necessary to do so and (b) if it is, then what their plan is for managing your hormones after removal. If a woman has not yet reached menopause, removing both ovaries is often called "surgical menopause" because it effectively puts a woman into menopause, with potentially uncomfortable side effects including hot flashes, vaginal dryness, and painful sex. Not all women experience these side effects, but it is important for you and your health care provider to communicate about these issues so that you can get the health care you need.

42. What to do if . . . you lose arousal just before orgasm and are sure it's "gone"

Wait it out! All too often, women are convinced that their sexual arousal is gone in the instant they think of something distracting (such as work that needs to get done, laundry that needs to be folded, or a lunch box that needs to be packed) or upsetting, such as a fight they had with their partner. A good bit of news is that our bodies are slow to catch up to the ways our minds race. Just because you think your sexual arousal is gone doesn't mean that it is. It takes as long as ten minutes for a woman's aroused body to become physically "unaroused" (for blood flow to move away from the genitals, etc.). So if you think it's gone, think again. And if you want it back, try to refocus your mind back to the sexy situation you're in. Try to use mindfulness techniques to focus on how the vibrator feels on your clitoris or how it tastes to kiss your partner. With an inhale, focus on how your partner's hair smells and with an out breath, focus on how it feels to touch his or her skin. Soon enough, you're likely to feel just as aroused as your body still is.

43. What to do if . . . he comes too quickly for you to orgasm

When two women have sex, sex doesn't necessarily end the second the first one of them has an orgasm. Put a man and a woman in bed, though, and things get tricky. Some couples are convinced that sex is over as soon as a man ejaculates. There is some truth to this, of course, if one is speaking strictly about penile-vaginal intercourse—but since when is penile-vaginal sex everything sex has to offer? If you're happy being pleasured another way, then turn to oral sex, sex toy play, or something else you find enjoyable or even orgasmic. If you prefer to have your orgasm during vaginal intercourse, you have a few options:

• **See if you're able to work together to prolong his orgasm and help him last longer.** Desensitizing condoms or even plain old thicker condoms may help him to last longer (see chapter 5 for additional tips on helping him last longer).

• **Spend more time in foreplay before letting him inside you.** Some women find that they orgasm more quickly when they are highly aroused. If this sounds like you, do something extra arousing before proceeding with intercourse, whether that's oral sex, dirty talk, tying your partner up, getting a good spanking, or having your breasts played with. Try to choose something that's highly arousing to you but perhaps only moderately arousing to him—after all, you want him to have fun but you don't want it to push him over the orgasmic edge too soon.

• **Don't let it stop you.** After men ejaculate, their penis loses some of its rigidity. However, many men still have enough "fullness" or hardness to pleasure their partner. Unfortunately, men sometimes feel like they need to pull out as soon as they ejaculate. Not so! (Unless, of course, you're using withdrawal as birth control, in which case he should have pulled out several moments before ejaculating: never, ever use withdrawal as a birth control method with a man who finds it difficult to control when and where he ejaculates.) If he keeps his somewhat-hard penis inside your vagina, you may still be able to have an orgasm. Don't give up!

Finally, try not to let the mismatched timing of your orgasms get in the way of pleasurable sex. Orgasm really isn't everything, and it would behoove you to help your partner feel good about his sexual performance rather than guilty or ashamed of it. All too often I hear from women who accuse men who come quickly of being "selfish" or "only in it for themselves" or who grow visibly upset or angry when he ejaculates. To the extent that you can stay calm and find another way to ask him to pleasure you, or to pleasure yourself, it may make your sex life together better and feel more rewarding.

44. What to do if . . . you're on the verge of orgasm but can't seem to get over the hump

Know that you're not alone. Millions of women try to have orgasms and find it very difficult to do so. It's generally thought that nearly every woman is physically capable of having orgasms. Some women seem to have an easier or more difficult time than others. It's not your fault if you find it difficult.

The process of learning to experience orgasm can take time, exploration, and a great deal of patience. One friend was certain she would never have an orgasm. It took her more than a decade of trying but one day she learned to. When she told me about the time it finally happened, she had tears in her eyes because she was so happy and had tried for so long. Although having an orgasm isn't important to everybody, it mattered to her a great deal and she had all but given up on the possibility.

Other women have an easier time learning to experience orgasm, alone or with a partner. Trying to experience orgasm alone during masturbation involves less pressure because no one is there asking "have you come yet?" Also, there's no internal pressure to have an orgasm and make your partner feel like they're great in bed. For these and other reasons (such as not being hesitant to display your "O" face during masturbation), exploring your sexual response in private is often a more effective way to learn to have an orgasm than trying with your partner.

Everyone is different, though, and some women feel very supported and encouraged by having their partner help them along the way. Some make it quite a fun affair and may use fantasy, new sex positions, porn, role-playing, relaxation, massage, or vibrators to enhance a woman's sexual arousal and chances of having an orgasm. If you have never had an orgasm and want to, try to focus on making your private and partnered sexual experiences pleasurable and relaxing. If you keep exploring things that you find pleasurable and arousing, you may ultimately hit upon something that helps you experience orgasm. Try to open your mind to the possibility that you may be most aroused, or most easily orgasmic, by ideas or fantasies that are different than you perhaps imagined. Some women and men are most aroused when fantasizing about group sex, sex with a stranger, or being very dominant or submissive. It's also the case that watching porn is sometimes highly exciting to women in ways that surprise them. And some women who consider themselves heterosexual and only have sex with men (and only want to have sex with men) find that fantasizing about being sexual with women is what sends them over the edge. Similarly, some women who identify as lesbian and only have sex with women are sometimes unexpectedly aroused by imagining having sex with a man (or multiple men).

The mind is a curious place and certainly nothing we've figured out. Why does one fantasy arouse someone to the point of orgasm yet disgust another person? We don't know. And why do many of us have sexual fantasies about things we would never want to do in real life? Again, there are many theories, but we simply don't know.

Finally, you might find it helpful to read *Becoming Orgasmic* by Julia Heiman, PhD, and Joseph LoPiccolo, PhD—a very good book that is entirely devoted to helping women learn to experience orgasm—or to meet with a sex therapist.

45. What to do if . . . you crave a multiple orgasm

Not long ago, one of my college students stayed after class to ask how to have multiple orgasms during intercourse with her boyfriend. She had previously had orgasms occasionally during intercourse but she couldn't reliably have them. She had experienced multiple orgasms only one time before, if I remember correctly, and she wanted to know what she could do to make them happen. I told her what I tell everyone else who asks this question—the advice worked for her—and what I'll now share with you.

Though a very small number of women have orgasms extremely easily and without trying to at all, most of us have to put in at least a little (or a lot of) effort to experience orgasm—if indeed we want to, and of course, orgasm isn't important to everyone. For most women who are into orgasm, though, we *try* to have orgasms; they don't just drop out of the sky. In my professional and personal experience, then, multiple orgasms seem to be helped by

- Being open to the possibility of them
- Going forward even when you think your arousal is done and gone, and
- Taking charge of your sensations

There is a lack of scientific research on the topic, but this has been true for me so I am basing this approach on my own experience—something that, as a scientist, I realize has its limitations. Your experience may be different.

In my case, after I learned to experience orgasm during intercourse, I felt very happy and satisfied with my experiences, just as I had before I learned to do so. I had heard from plenty of women who found it difficult to have orgasms and thus knew that I was fortunate that I had not only learned to orgasm during intercourse but that I had practiced it enough that I could do it reliably. For the longest time, though, I didn't try to have multiple orgasms. I was truly content with one, just as I had previously been content with none.

In my experience, multiple orgasms had often been talked about loudly and openly by women who almost seemed to be bragging about it, as if having an orgasm was a competition. Or else I heard about it from men who also seemed to be boasting about the tons and tons of orgasms they were giving women all over the world. I don't know if it's just me or if others feel this way, but all that bragging left a bad taste in my mouth, and I guess I didn't want to be one of "those women." I had experienced multiple orgasms during masturbation and never really saw the need to do so during intercourse. Wasn't one orgasm enough? It was for me.

Then I met an interesting person who changed my thinking. I had been asked to give a sex talk to a small group of women who were friends with each other. They had flown to be together for a girls' weekend and hired me to travel to the city, drink wine with them, and talk with them about sex. In a beautiful suite at a luxury hotel, I sat with these women, who ranged in age from their early forties to their early fifties. While we were talking about orgasm, they started asking each other about it. One of the friends turned to another—a sophisticated and conservative-looking woman in her early fifties—and asked her point-blank if she had multiple orgasms. Blushing, she said (almost reluctantly) that she did. Her friends grew excited in the way that groups of girlfriends do, and they asked her for more details. After all, as it turned out, none of the rest of them had had this experience. The woman shared a few details: She and her husband, being empty nesters, had more time for sex than they had earlier in life. Sometimes, she said, they would pour glasses of wine, retreat into the bedroom, and make love. She would have an orgasm or two and then they would stop and talk, drink some more wine, and continue with their lovemaking, with more orgasms to come here and there.

There was something about this woman's approach to multiple orgasms that interested and even moved me. When her friends asked about her experience, she was happy to share with them. But she never seemed to be bragging about her sex life. If anything, it sometimes seemed that she didn't want to tell her friends how fantastic her sex life and marriage were, lest they walk away feeling less positive about their own. She didn't seem to see sex or orgasm as a competition or anything that made her better than her friends. I appreciated that about her, and I began to wonder if I was capable of multiple orgasms and, if I was, how that would feel for me. It may sound silly, but it was the first time I had imagined that one could be both multiply orgasmic and noncompetitive.

When I returned home to my partner, the next time we had sex and I experienced an orgasm, I secretly decided that I wanted to try to have a second one. I didn't tell him I was trying, I just focused on my own sensations and went for it. To my surprise, it worked—and of course he was delighted when it happened. This was an important experience for me personally (because it taught me how to have multiple orgasms during intercourse, which I experience very differently from orgasms during masturbation). But it was also an important experience for me professionally. It reinforced for me the power of the mind and the value of mentally opening oneself to an experience. This does not mean that all one has to do is be "open" to multiple orgasms, but it may mean that for some women it's an important part of the picture. As a sex educator, I find this valuable information to share with others (even though this is the first time I have ever shared my own experience with multiple orgasm with others—again, I've worried about coming off as competitive or "braggy").

As I mentioned earlier, it can also be helpful to orgasm if you keep going with sex even after you think your arousal is gone. After a woman has her first orgasm, she may think that's it and that her body is ready to return to its unaroused pre-sex state. Yet her body is likely still physically aroused, which is a great place to be if she's interested in going forward and trying to have multiple orgasms.

Taking charge of your own sensations is also critical. You might try asking your partner to stay still for a few moments during sex while you control the sensation. If your partner is a man, have him stay still while you squeeze your vagina around his penis. Try moving your hips in ways that stimulate your vagina and clitoris in ways that feel good to you. If you're trying for multiple orgasms during oral sex, try to direct your partner's tongue by gently adjusting his head, or else give him or her verbal directions ("slower" or "more gentle" or "put a finger in") to help along the way. Given that, as I mentioned earlier, there is a lack of scientific research on multiple orgasm, we don't know much about how many women have them or in what contexts (for example, with vaginal orgasm, masturbation, oral sex); however, I hope that if you're interested in trying to experience multiple orgasm, this is a helpful start.

Finally, know that multiple orgasms don't always mean "better" orgasms or stronger ones. Sometimes women who experience multiple orgasms will say that the first one feels the best or strongest. Other times, on any given day, the second or fifth one does. They're all different from each other and unique in their own ways.

46. What to do if . . . you want a simultaneous orgasm

Not all couples can have simultaneous orgasm. For one thing, many women and a small proportion of men find it difficult if not impossible to experience orgasm. Also, most women and a sizable number of men find it difficult to control the timing of their orgasm. It's no wonder that an important characteristic of many porn actors involves their ability to ejaculate when the director says "Go!" (whereas many porn actresses simply fake it).

Honestly, I wish people didn't feel so much that they need to orgasm together. Aside from knowing that your partner probably isn't looking at your awkward "O" face because they're too busy making their own awkward "O" face, I don't personally see a great deal of benefit from it.

But if you absolutely are into having simultaneous orgasms with your partner, here are my thoughts. As far as I can tell, it seems that there are two types of men with whom simultaneous orgasm seems an easier feat. Men with premature ejaculation, if they can hold out long enough, may be so easily excitable that when you experience orgasm, they feel like they can finally "let go" and experience orgasm too. That's one type. The other type of man is the rare kind who can come when and where he wants to. If you want him to come quickly, he can. If you want him to wait longer so sex lasts for a long time or so you have a greater chance of one or more orgasms, he can do that too. He has what we scientists call "good ejaculatory control." There is no Olympic competition for such men, but it truly is quite a skill that, I think, is helped by both natural ability (genetics) and practice.

If you're a woman whose partner is also a woman, then unless one of you finds it extremely easy to orgasm whenever she wants to, it might be tough to time your orgasms together that precisely. Similarly, if you're a woman whose male partner has delayed ejaculation and they find it very difficult to ejaculate, then unless you can orgasm with the snap of your fingers, whenever you want, it may be difficult to align your orgasms together.

Which is why I say that if you want simultaneous orgasms and it happens, then great. And if not, try to focus on something else. There are so many wonderful parts of sex—there are sexy sights, smells, tastes, and a great deal of connection and fun to be had—so try not to let this one issue keep you from enjoying the rest of your time between the sheets.

Sex Smarts Quiz

1. Women who participated in my study about orgasm-induced exercise described having orgasms during
    a. Yoga
    b. Bike riding
    c. Running
    d. All of the above
2. Compared to other women, those whose clitoris is closer to their urethra may be ____ likely to experience orgasm during sex.
    a. More
    b. Less
    c. Equally
3. Women have reported experiencing orgasms during
    a. Breastfeeding
    b. Sleep
    c. Childbirth
    d. All of the above

Answers
    1. d
    2. a
    3. d

Chapter 5
Erections and Ejaculation: Your Road Map to Better, What-to-Expect Sex

I f you've ever found yourself in the middle of an exciting sexual encounter only to find that the man's penis won't get hard or stay hard (or he comes very quickly)—no matter what you do to it—join the club. Most men experience erection difficulties at some point in their lives. And a sizable number of men—as many as 20 percent—will experience moderate to severe erectile dysfunction (ED) in which they have difficulty getting or keeping an erection in most circumstances (both with masturbation and partnered sex) over a period of time.[1] Ejaculation difficulties are common too, with as many as 20 to 30 percent of men experiencing premature ejaculation and a smaller number of men finding it difficult, if not impossible, to ejaculate during sex.[2]

The penis cannot be 100 percent controlled, no matter how easily excited or aroused a man feels. Yet we women who have sex with men often feel as if our male partner's penis is our responsibility—that it's our job to get their penis hard and keep it hard or else we've done something wrong. To that I say, "Poppycock!"

Still, I understand how and why it is that women feel this way. Men often tell their partners that they're hard *because of them* ("Look what you did to me!" they might say, staring down at their erection, suggesting that their partner is so hot, attractive, or sexy that it made them hard). Or a man might come quickly and then tell his partner that he came so fast because she's so hot or because she squeezed her vaginal muscles during intercourse (thus stimulating his penis). This certainly happens. But while it's true that men commonly get erections from looking at, fantasizing about, or being touched by a sexual partner, the lack of an erection doesn't necessarily mean that a man is not interested, excited, or anything less than totally turned on. Penises don't always work as planned.

Dozens of factors can influence a man's erections and ejaculation and not all of them have to do with how attracted he feels to his partner. As just a few examples, a man's erections may be influenced by

- Hormones
- His age
- How he feels, emotionally, about his partner
- Performance anxiety
- Sadness or grief
- The temperature in the room
- His relationship with his partner
- Medical conditions
- Prescription drugs
- Cigarette smoking
- Over-the-counter medications
- Cardiovascular health
- Recreational drugs
- Work stress
- Alcohol use
- Feeling rested or tired
- Feeling relaxed or stressed
- How a condom feels on his penis
- Worries about getting or giving an STI
- Feeling worried or excited about the possibility that his partner might become pregnant
- Time of day
- Worry about hurting one's partner
- How long it's been since he last ejaculated
  ... and much, much more.

Most of the above can also influence a man's ejaculation.

In spite of the many factors that can contribute to a man's penis being as hard as a rock or as soft as a cloth, men's erections are often treated as though they are completely simple and easy to operate. A common myth is that men can control their erections and when they ejaculate, when in reality they rarely have much say about either. This can feel distressing for many men. After all, if we women feel aroused but our bodies don't cooperate—meaning we end up with a not-so-wet vagina—we can always add lubricant (or, in a pinch, saliva) to make sex go more smoothly. Sex can proceed as usual. When men's bodies don't cooperate, though, men often feel like failures, as if they've done something wrong. Without an erection, many men feel like sex is a no-go and they may feel extra pressure if their partner tries to regain their erection by using their hands or mouth to desperately bring it back to life.

ERECTION AND EJACULATION BASICS

In chapter 2, we talked a little about erections and how they happen. Physical touching or mental stimulation (fantasy: exciting or arousing thoughts) can stimulate messages to the nerves in a man's penis. The penis then relaxes its blood vessels, allowing blood to flow more easily and fully into the penis. As the penis becomes larger, pressure constricts a vein that would otherwise let the blood flow right back out of the penis. The result is more blood flowing into the penis than out of it, "trapping" the blood in the two spongy tissues called the corpora cavernosa.

Ejaculation is triggered in a somewhat mysterious way (scientists don't fully understand it) when men reach a certain level of physical or mental excitement that pushes them over the edge. There are two phases to men's ejaculation. The first phase is called **emission:** this is when the vas deferens helps move sperm from the testes to the back of a man's urethra through a series of contractions (men can often feel these contractions). There, at the back of the urethra, the sperm get mixed in with fluids from a man's prostate gland and seminal vesicles, creating a melting pot of fluids that are ultimately called "semen" when combined. The second phase is called **expulsion** and it's when the semen comes out of the penis, typically in spurts. Once this part of the process begins, there's no stopping it—which is a key difference between men's orgasms and women's orgasms.

Speaking of orgasm, it should be noted that men's ejaculation and orgasm are two different experiences. Although the vast majority of men experience them as one and the same (meaning that when they orgasm, they also ejaculate and when they ejaculate, they also orgasm), some men can or do experience them as separate events. There are men who ejaculate without experiencing any accompanying feelings of pleasure or euphoria that are commonly thought of as orgasm. Also, some men teach themselves to experience the excitement of orgasm without ejaculating (this is sometimes taught as part of tantric sex workshops). I've heard from a number of men who have taught themselves to separate orgasms from ejaculation. Some tried it out of curiosity but thought that, in the end, it wasn't anything particularly pleasurable for them ("A lot of work for nothing," said one platonic friend of mine who learned to do this). Other men greatly enjoy having orgasms while delaying their actual ejaculation. Like most areas of sex, it seems to be a matter of individual preference.

IT'S GONE. NOW WHAT?

Men's erections (much like women's orgasms) tend to thrive in situations of relaxation—not pressure. If you've ever felt pressured to have an orgasm by a partner who tries and tries and keeps asking "Did you come yet?" then you may be able to identify with men's feelings of frustration or irritation during sex. You may have even faked orgasm to get him to stop asking if you've come yet or to help him feel good about his sexual performance (some men fake too, and for the same reasons). Many men feel similarly when their partner keeps trying to make their penis hard again. Even if they're not asking about the state of their partner's penis ("Are you hard yet? How about now?"), the pressure is there.

When a man loses an erection, rather than focus all your energy on his penis, try to focus your energy elsewhere. This can take the pressure off him to get an erection. Try to give your attention to other body parts and to ways of being sexual that don't "require" an erect penis. You might try

• Moving his hands to your breasts or butt

- Turning him over onto his stomach for an erotic massage, during which you kiss his neck, massage his back, and use your hands to stroke his butt and inner thighs
- Asking for oral sex, either verbally or nonverbally (such as by crawling into a position in which your vulva is near his face)
- Getting out a vibrator and asking him to use it on you
- Watching porn together
- Reading sexy poetry together
- Asking him to tie you up and please you in unanticipated ways (maybe even blindfolded)
- Kissing, and kissing some more

If he gets another erection and you two decide to "use it" somehow, such as for vaginal sex, oral sex, anal sex, or mutual masturbation, then enjoy. Just because he gets an erection, however, doesn't mean you should pounce on it as if that's the one thing you have been hoping for. If he becomes erect, give his penis some time. The more the two of you can build his arousal, the better chance he will have at keeping his erection going. If he doesn't get another erection, that's okay too. If he has recently ejaculated (whether with you or during masturbation), it could be hours before he can get a very firm and reliable erection again. It happens.

HOW ERECTIONS THRIVE

Common myths about men suggest that they're mainly into casual sex and only "settle" for sex with a long-term love because it's expected of them. Reality tells a different story. The vast majority of my male college students write their papers about the enormous value they place on sex within the context of a relationship. It's not unusual for them to write about how much they enjoyed casual hookups until they finally found a girlfriend and realized that sex with emotional components could be a far more enriching and exciting experience for them. If anything, my male college students often feel misunderstood and stereotyped and say that they wish more women realized that men are people too, and want to love and be loved just as much as the next person (and yes, they crave sex too).

It was no surprise, then, to find in our National Survey of Sexual Health and Behavior that adult men were less likely to report erectile problems during sex with a relationship partner (such as a girlfriend or wife) compared to sex with a casual partner. Because men's erections thrive when they're feeling comfortable and relaxed, it makes sense that they'd be more likely to have stronger, easier erections with someone they know well and around whom they can be themselves. After all, men aren't some alien species who only want sex sex sex. They also want to be held, to be loved, and to feel comfortable when they're stripped naked and in bed with another person.

THE CARE AND FEEDING OF A MAN'S ERECTIONS

Comfortable relationships and relaxing, low-pressure sex are just some of the factors that can enhance men's sexual response. Another has to do with the things we all do day in and day out: that is, how we eat, exercise, and generally care for ourselves.

In a 2011 study published in the *Archives of Internal Medicine*, researchers from the Mayo Clinic analyzed data from six clinical trials in four countries.[3] They found that men who made positive changes to how they ate and exercised were able to significantly improve their cardiovascular health and erectile function. To keep your partner's penis in tip-top shape, encourage him to eat foods such as those that make up a Mediterranean diet (for example, fruits, vegetables, legumes, and walnuts). If he's able to exercise, encourage moderate to rigorous exercise upwards of three hours per week—not all at one time, of course, but spread throughout the week. (Of course, he should always check in with his health care provider before starting a physical exercise program.) These kinds of lifestyle factors may help him live a longer, healthy life with more opportunities for sexual sharing. They also build on previous research that has found that smoking cigarettes negatively affects men's sexual function, including their erectile function. The bottom line is that lifestyle factors such as sleep, exercise, not smoking, and eating well matter to our sexual health as well as our heart health.

THE REFRACTORY PERIOD

Along with getting an erection in the first place, many people are curious about how a man goes about getting a second erection after ejaculating. Men's post-ejaculation refractory time (PERT)—commonly called the "refractory period" (the time it takes to get another firm erection after an ejaculation)—is not well understood.[4] Here's what we know: Men commonly report that they feel unable to get another solid erection soon after they ejaculate. Some men notice that their refractory period changes with age; they will often say that their refractory period was short as a teenager or young adult (meaning that they could go over and over again) and grew longer with age. Other men don't notice an age-related change to their refractory period and, even in their sixties and seventies can repeatedly get erections and ejaculate in the span of an hour or two.

It is interesting that scientists don't understand what controls a man's refractory period even though several studies have tried to examine the issue. Results are similarly mixed on whether or not medications make a difference: some research has found that sildenafil (Viagra) can shorten a man's refractory period, helping him get another erection soon after ejaculating. Other research has found that taking sildenafil has no effect on the refractory period.

While scientists continue to learn more on the topic, what can you do at home? Perhaps the most important approach is to respect your partner's experience. Some men can get another erection quickly after ejaculating. Others cannot. It can also change from day to day. If you want to keep being sexual with him but he cannot get another erection, try to expand your ideas of sex and do something that doesn't require an erection (make use of each other's fingers, tongues, mouths, or a sex toy).

LASTING LONGER: TWO TECHNIQUES YOU SHOULD KNOW

In many ways, women are grassroots sex educators. I don't know if it's in our nature or how we're raised (it's probably a bit of each), but some research suggests that women feel responsible for being the ones to make their sex lives more exciting. This is also probably why so many women write and/or read sex books like this one. Of course, men need to be responsible for doing their share to make sex better too. And to the extent that we all keep learning about sex and talking about it with each other, we can all have a better shot at more wonderful sex. Many men feel reluctant to talk about their health—or their sex lives—in frank ways with their friends or doctors. That means it's often the case that women who learn about sex end up sharing what they learn with their partners.

If your partner comes more quickly than he'd like to (remember, it's common with about 20 to 30 percent of men experiencing premature ejaculation) and would like to learn how to better control when he ejaculates, share these two techniques with him. It's best if he practices them first during masturbation on his own. Once he feels he has them down, you might want to try them together, with you kissing him while he masturbates himself or, eventually, with you being the one to stimulate him.

The techniques are called the Stop-Start and Squeeze Techniques and men have been using them for decades in and out of sex therapy. Here's how they work:

The Stop-Start Technique

A man begins this by stimulating his penis in whatever way he normally does during masturbation. As he builds sexual arousal and a stronger erection, he will want to stop all stimulation to his penis just before "the point of no return" (when he will ejaculate no matter what happens). After he stops all stimulation, he can then wait several seconds or longer until his arousal slightly decreases while still maintaining his erection. Then he can start stimulating his penis again and repeating the cycle several times before finally letting himself ejaculate.

The Squeeze Technique

This starts out in an identical fashion as the Stop-Start Technique. The main difference is that instead of stopping all stimulation to the penis, the man gently squeezes the head of his penis to help decrease his arousal and excitement before restarting stimulation. The cycle repeats several times before allowing ejaculation to occur.

Both techniques are meant to help men identify the points at which they start to become highly excited and close to ejaculating. When they learn to identify the bodily sensations that lead up to this point, they can then adjust their masturbation or partnered sex so that they can back off a little and eventually learn to last longer without ejaculating. It can take weeks or months for a man to notice significant improvement in his ejaculatory control.

Once men feel comfortable with one of these techniques during masturbation and have made some progress at lasting longer on their own, they may want to try it with their partner (that's you!). Personally, I think the Stop-Start Technique is easiest to transfer to sex with a partner because all it requires is stopping sexual stimulation; there's no squeezing involved. This is particularly helpful for intercourse. During vaginal intercourse, in an effort to last longer some men simply stop moving for several seconds until they are able to experience a decrease in sensation. Other times, if a man feels he is close to ejaculating, he might pull his penis out of his partner's body and then give it a few seconds before resuming intercourse. He might even suggest switching positions to one that stimulates his penis less directly. Some men, for example, find rear entry positions (in which they are entering their partner's vagina from behind) to be very physically and mentally stimulating and they may not be able to last long in that position. They may be able to last longer in missionary or woman on top, however (men vary, so ask your partner how different positions feel for him).

Notes from the Premature Ejaculation Trenches

I'm always a bit sad to hear from men and women who believe that premature ejaculation necessarily makes for bad sex. I don't believe this to be the case at all. Does it make for sex that is different from sex with a man who can last for hours if he wants to? Of course. But different is just different; it's not necessarily any better or worse.

Case in point. I once dated a man who had a lifelong history of experiencing premature ejaculation. We never timed it, but my best guess is that he typically came within thirty seconds to two minutes of penetration (which was significantly quicker than other people I had dated). Yet the sex wasn't bad. In fact, it was very good. I think there were several reasons for this. First, we had an extremely emotionally close relationship and a great deal of chemistry. Some research studies have found that the psychological component of sex is often more important to sexual satisfaction than things like penis size or technique (or, I would add, how long a couple spends having intercourse). And while he had previously felt a great deal of shame and embarrassment about coming quickly with past partners, I recognized early on that I wanted to change that. After all, shame and embarrassment don't bring a lot of good energy to the bedroom whereas pride and confidence do. I made it a personal mission to be kind, supportive, and complimentary to him about his penis and sexual technique so that he would come to see his body as I did (as something sexy rather than shameful).

Together, we also looked on the bright side: while he wasn't able to last as long as he wanted, he was able to get a second (or third) erection relatively soon after he ejaculated, which meant that we were able to have sex again later on if we wanted to—and we often did. Further, we simply enjoyed being in bed together talking, reading, laughing, and kissing. In addition, rather than view his premature ejaculation as a bad thing, I chose to look at it as a challenge: if I wanted to reach orgasm during intercourse, I had to learn to do so more quickly (which I eventually taught myself to do).

When I teach human sexuality classes to college students, I don't share stories from my personal sex life. Yet I often feel that personal stories have the potential to add significant value to learning, particularly for such a taboo topic as sexuality. I hope that because I shared this experience, some of you will walk away with a new perspective on premature ejaculation. If your partner comes very quickly, try to imagine a more positive way to look at your situation. Spending more time together in ways that help you laugh, dance, joke, share deep feelings, and enjoy each other's company may help you build such a strong chemistry or closeness that the length of time it takes for him to ejaculate simply stops mattering to you. To judge an entire relationship by the speed with which semen flows out of a man's penis seems a waste to me, especially when there is so much pleasure to be had if only you can open your eyes to it. Men often carry around a great deal of embarrassment and shame related to how their penis works (or doesn't work) and how long (or how quickly) it takes them to ejaculate. Try to help your partner feel positively about his sexuality and you may end up with a better sex life for it.

OLD HABITS DIE HARD

Coming too quickly isn't the only ejaculation issue men experience, although it is the most common. A minority of men take a very long time to ejaculate (called "delayed ejaculation") and wish they could come more quickly.

In his book *The New Male Sexuality*, the late sex therapist Bernie Zilbergeld noted that a number of his patients with delayed ejaculation tended to rely on uncommon masturbation techniques.[5] In my years working as a sex columnist and sex educator, I, too, have heard from a number of men who find it difficult or impossible to ejaculate and probably 90 percent of them describe masturbating in ways that are different from many other men's techniques. Specifically, many men with delayed ejaculation will tell me that ever since childhood or adolescence they have masturbated by rubbing their penis against the carpet or their bed or, in some cases, using a very strong vibrating device (such as a vibrating back massager) for masturbation.

Like many scientists who study sex, I don't know which came first. Do these men have a difficult time ejaculating because they've trained their bodies to respond to things like rubbing against a carpet or bed (and then when they go to have vaginal sex, oral sex, or anal sex, it just doesn't feel the same)? Or did they start masturbating against the carpet or bed (or with a vibrator) because they first tried using their hands and found that it didn't work out, perhaps because their genitals aren't as sensitive as other men's genitals? We don't know. I do know, though, that many of the men I've talked to have been able to learn to ejaculate more quickly and easily during oral sex, vaginal sex, anal sex, or masturbation. Here's how:

I ask them to consider trying to vary their masturbation routine at home. I suggest that they avoid the carpet or bed routine for several days, allowing them to build sexual tension and arousal. Then, when they masturbate, I encourage them to try it with a dry hand one day and a well-lubricated hand the next time several days later. I encourage them to use sexual fantasy occasionally and sexual materials (whatever they find exciting, such as books, stories, audio CDs or podcasts, or porn videos) another time. By varying their masturbation routine, many men are able to eventually train their body to ejaculate in new ways—and, at some point, to do so with a partner as well. Of course, a new masturbation routine takes time and it isn't a quick fix. Having a caring, supportive, and patient partner is helpful as well (and so is sex therapy, particularly for long-standing cases of delayed ejaculation).

For Your Library

If your partner has erectile, ejaculatory, or performance anxiety problems or concerns, I would also recommend that you read *The Sexual Male: Problems and Solutions* and/or *The New Male Sexuality* together. These are two of my favorite books about men's sexuality and many of my students and column readers have found them helpful as well. Add them to your library, read them together, and—most importantly—talk about them together.

— Making It Easy —

47. What to do if . . . your partner comes lightning fast

The number-one rule when dealing with a man who comes quickly is to be kind and compassionate. If you're thinking to yourself, "Who wouldn't be kind?", let me tell you who: many of the people I hear from. It's not that they're bad people. However, false myths about men's sexuality suggest that they should all naturally have a magical ability to last as long as men in porn films or Hollywood movies. These myths contribute to many men feeling ashamed and embarrassed that they cannot last longer. Also, many women who take some time to reach orgasm blame men who come quickly for their lack of orgasm ("I need at least fifteen minutes of sex before I can have an orgasm," they might say, "and when you come that fast, I don't get a chance to come"). I've heard far too many women say, "He's just selfish!"—as if their partner purposely chose to come quickly or leave them feeling sexually frustrated.

Condoms to Help Him Last Longer

These condoms—which are often called "performance condoms" or "desensitizing condoms"—contain small amounts of substances such as benzocaine or lidocaine that slightly decrease sensation in a man's penis, thus helping him last longer. If you go this route, keep in mind that this is a short-term strategy, meaning that it will only work when he uses it. Also, it's extra important that the condom is applied correctly. If a man puts this type of condom on inside out, the numbing sensation could get in your vagina or anus (depending on what kind of sex you're having), which may lead to irritation or a "numb" vagina or anus. A few other notes of caution: Some men may react so strongly to the desensitizing substances that they feel more numb than expected, and they may lose their erections (not exactly what's intended). In addition, a small percentage of men may be sensitive or allergic to the desensitizing substances, which can lead to a rash or genital irritation. These can be great sexual enhancement tools but they're not for everyone.

Just as most women don't purposely take a long time to orgasm, the roughly one-quarter to one-third of men who come more quickly than they'd like aren't speeding it up on purpose. It's a rare man who can come exactly when he wants to and adjust his timing (coming more quickly or lasting longer) to please his partner.

If you and your partner are both into the idea of him lasting longer, try to be supportive of him learning how, which can take time. There are several strategies to try including

• **Using desensitizing condoms.** Available in many drugstores and online, these condoms work by using desensitizing substances (included in a lubricant that lines the inside of the condom) to slightly decrease sensation in a man's penis, thus helping him to last a minute or two longer during sex—and in some cases, a bit longer (see sidebar on page 127).

• **Practicing the Stop-Start and/or Squeeze Techniques.** Detailed earlier in this chapter, these two techniques help some men create long-term changes with their ejaculatory control.

• **Relaxation strategies.** For many men, performance anxiety or other forms of stress and anxiety contribute to, or cause, rapid and uncontrolled ejaculation. Deep breathing, meditation, mindfulness, and other relaxation techniques can help men learn to relax during sex, enjoy their bodily sensations, and experience more pleasurable—yet controllable—sexual experiences.

• **Practicing yoga.** Several studies have found that men who practice yoga often experience improvements in their sexual function, including better ejaculatory control, perhaps due to enhanced focus and attention on their bodily sensations combined with improvement in their ability to relax.[6]

• **Prescription medications.** Some medications, including some prescription antidepressant medications, have been tested and found to be effective at helping men last longer.[7] This is often considered a "last resort" strategy for rapid ejaculation, with relaxation techniques and the Stop-Start Technique being among the earlier recommended strategies, but it's a good one for many men. Ask your health care provider for more information.

It Takes a (Massive) Village

Women are more likely to become pregnant when they have sex with a man who has at least sixty million sperm per milliliter. While it's widely known that there are millions of sperm swimming around in a man's semen, stop and think about it: the 2011 population of New York City is just over eight million people. Multiply that by about $7^{1}/_{2}$ and you have the number of sperm in just one milliliter of semen to have the best pregnancy odds. No worries, though: each testicle makes several million new sperm *every hour*, so there should be plenty to go around.

---

48. What to do if . . . your partner can't have an orgasm during vaginal or oral sex

A small percentage of men—probably fewer than 5 percent—find it extremely difficult or even impossible to ejaculate. Sometimes this is specific to a certain sex act: a man may be able to ejaculate during vaginal sex but not oral sex. Other times, it's the difference between partnered sex and masturbation. For example, some men find it easy enough to ejaculate when they masturbate but when they're having sex with a partner, they can't ejaculate no matter what they try (vaginal sex, oral sex, mutual masturbation, etc.). And then there are men who find it difficult or impossible to ejaculate in any situation, masturbation or partnered.

Men who take a very long time to ejaculate, say forty-five to sixty minutes, are sometimes considered to have "delayed ejaculation," meaning they can do it, but it takes a while. Men who find that they are unable to ejaculate in certain circumstances may be described as experiencing "inhibited ejaculation."

Considering that these are relatively uncommon sexual difficulties, they are among the more common questions I get: perhaps because there is so little information available about delayed and inhibited ejaculation (erectile dysfunction and premature ejaculation are more common and thus more widely talked and written about). When I write sex columns about this issue, emails often flood my mailbox from men who tell me that they, too, find it difficult to ejaculate and thanking me for helping them to not feel so alone or "weird."

There are many reasons why a man may experience delayed or inhibited ejaculation. Some men seem to have genitals that are not very sensitive and that may require significant stimulation in order to experience orgasm and ejaculation. In some cases, these men find it easier to ejaculate when they watch porn and/or use a vibrator during masturbation or sex; very intense vibrators such as the Hitachi Magic Wand or Acuvibe are preferred by some men with whom I've spoken. Other times, psychological characteristics such as a fear of letting go or losing control are at the root of a man's delayed or inhibited ejaculation. It's also the case that men who can experience orgasm during masturbation or oral sex, but not during vaginal sex, are sometimes afraid of getting their female partner pregnant. Truly, there are a number of reasons why some men find it difficult to ejaculate, including some medical conditions. For these reasons, men who find it difficult to ejaculate and who want to try to change this should see a health care provider, who can rule out medical conditions and medication-related side effects. Often, they can also benefit from seeing a sex therapist who can help provide suggestions for ways to adjust sex for greater stimulation (for example, vibrator use). A sex therapist can also help the man and his partner examine the various psychological aspects of delayed or inhibited ejaculation in ways that might be effective.

Know, too, that delayed ejaculation isn't necessarily a bad thing. Men whose partners find it uncomfortable or painful to have sex for as long as it takes for him to come would be wise to change sex up so that the partner doesn't feel "burdened" to keep going until the man ejaculates. If he can come during masturbation, then the couple may find it more pleasurable to spend however long they want to during vaginal or oral sex and then, when they're ready to be done, switch to masturbation. That way, he can ejaculate without causing pain or discomfort to his partner by repeatedly thrusting in and out in an effort to ejaculate. On the other hand, if the man's partner enjoys spending a long time during sex, then having a partner who takes a long time to ejaculate may feel like they've hit the jackpot. Much of sex has to do with one's perspective and if you *see* it as a good thing, it may end up *feeling* like a good thing.

Finally, men who are unable to ejaculate and who want to get their partner pregnant have added motivation to resolve this issue. After all, if they can't get sperm out of their body, then they won't stand a chance at impregnating their partner. Men in this situation may find it helpful to see a urologist or a fertility specialist who can help with other solutions to this dilemma, such as providing prostate stimulation or intense vibrator stimulation to help him ejaculate, procure sperm, and perhaps use it to perform in vitro fertilization. Where there's a will, there's a way.

49. What to do if . . . he has erection problems when he uses condoms

Most men will experience erectile problems at some point or another; that's a given. Men cannot perfectly control their penises or "will themselves" to get or keep an erection whenever they want. Erectile difficulties, then, are a fact of life, and something we would all do better to accept rather than feel anxious or upset about when they happen.

Some men are prone to erection problems in specific circumstances, such as when they use condoms.[8] It's not well understood why this happens to some men when they use condoms and not others. Researchers have long speculated on this, wondering if some men have condom-related erection difficulties because they're nervous about using a condom, more likely to be having sex with someone they don't know well, or because the condom doesn't fit or feel comfortable on their penis. It may even be that men are simply distracted by the act of putting a condom on their penis, and instead of focusing on the many things that would strengthen their erection (such as looking at or touching their sexy partner) they are instead having to focus on opening a condom package, carefully removing a condom, and putting it on their penis correctly.

If your partner has erectile difficulties with condom use, don't let that stand in the way of having safer sex. This is no reason to throw condoms by the wayside; you *can* work it out together. Tackle the issue head-on by talking about it. Offer to brainstorm viable solutions together. You might offer to put the condom on your partner's penis yourself so that he can focus on kissing and touching you and checking you out, while you focus on the mechanics of getting the condom out and on him. Once the condom is on his penis, put some water-based lubricant on your fingers and seductively stroke his condom-covered penis, spreading the lube up and down his shaft. Not only might this feel arousing to him (and thus help to firm up his erection), but the lubricant will also likely make penetration more comfortable and pleasurable once intercourse begins.

It's also the case that some men truly need a larger or differently sized condom. If your partner is larger than average, then look for a larger than average-sized condom such as Trojan Magnum XL. The Trojan Ecstasy line of condoms is also worth looking into. The shaft of Ecstasy condoms is baggier and shaped almost like a baseball, with more room for larger-sized men and for men who simply want enhanced sensation during sex (baggier condoms may enhance sensation because they're less likely to constrict the nerve endings of a man's penis). In one independent condom survey I conducted for *Men's Health* magazine, a number of men indicated that they felt the Ecstasy condoms made sex feel more natural and as if they weren't even using a condom (even though they were). Pleasure Plus and Inspiral condom brands also offer a little more room in their design. Finally, although these condom types are roomier in the shaft and/or head, the base of the condom is still snug in order to stay on securely during sex. No one wants a condom to slip off during sex!

50. What to do if . . . he has erection problems with pretty much any type of sex

A man who has persistent erectile problems should always mention this to a health care provider who can then examine him, run any necessary tests, and help determine the likely cause of his erectile difficulties or erectile dysfunction. If his ED is physical in nature, then a prescription medication may help. However, there is another important reason that men should mention erectile problems to their health care provider and that is because sometimes such problems are among the early symptoms of cardiovascular disease, such as heart or circulatory problems. Some research has found that ED may precede coronary artery disease by as many as two to five years, meaning that ED may be an important early warning sign to notice rather than ignore.

A man might also be referred to a sex therapist to help manage his erectile difficulties. After all, many young and/or healthy men have erectile difficulties that are caused or made worse by performance anxiety: the feeling of stress or anxiety about being a "good enough lover" and pleasing one's partner. Sex therapy has helped millions of men and their partners overcome or otherwise manage erectile problems.

51. What to do if . . . no semen comes out his penis when he has an orgasm

When a man feels as though he's having an orgasm but little to no semen spurts out of his penis (a "dry orgasm"), he's often said to be experiencing retrograde ejaculation. This is when semen goes backward into a man's bladder rather than ejaculating through the urethra and out of the penis. It's a relatively uncommon condition but when it happens, many men are taken aback and feel alone or unusual, so it's important to talk about it so that men and their partners don't feel this way. There is nothing necessarily bad or unhealthy about retrograde ejaculation and it doesn't bother everyone who experiences it. In fact, some men and their partners like that there's no "mess" or "cleanup" involved in their orgasms.

On the other hand, some men and their partners are turned on by the look or feel of ejaculation and may wish for a fix to the situation so that they can experience their own at-home, in-bed geyser in action. For some men and their partners, retrograde ejaculation becomes a fertility issue. If they wish to become pregnant, they need the sperm to get out of the penis, and thus they need to get him to ejaculate. Men who would like to kick their ejaculation into gear should let their health care provider know that they have been experiencing dry orgasms. If retrograde ejaculation has been caused by medications (such as some medications used to treat hypertension or depression), then stopping those medications—under the advice or supervision of a health care provider—may correct the problem.

Sometimes prescription medications are used to help a man to ejaculate out of his penis (these medications often work by helping keep the bladder neck muscle closed so that semen doesn't enter the bladder and instead leaves the body via ejaculation). In some cases, such as when retrograde ejaculation is caused by past surgical complications, medications may not be effective. If a man and his partner wish to become pregnant, a fertility specialist may be able to help recover semen from a man's bladder, process it, and use the sperm to help impregnate his partner. If your partner has dry orgasms and you want to become pregnant together, encourage him to see his health care provider, as in most cases some form of treatment is successful and men are able to impregnate their partners.

What Are You Swallowing, Anyway?

As mentioned in chapter 2, semen is composed of fluids from several different parts of a man's body. Most of the fluids (about 65 to 75 percent by volume) come from the seminal vesicles. About 25 to 30 percent comes from the prostate gland, and only a small amount comes from the Cowper's glands, which are two small pea-sized glands near the inside base of the penis (the fluid is the pre-ejaculatory fluid, also called "pre-cum"). Among these fluids are said to be proteins, vitamin C, flavins, prostaglandins, fructose, potassium, sodium, zinc, and more. I've seen calorie estimates that range from five to twenty-five calories per "serving" but no good data on actual figures. Rest assured, though, that the calories in semen have nothing on cheese fries. If you enjoy swallowing (and your partner doesn't have an STI), don't let calories stand in your way. And if you're not into it, there's no need to do it. There are many pleasurable ways to enjoy oral sex and swallowing isn't in the cards for everyone.

52. What to do if . . . it no longer feels good to him when he ejaculates

Men who ejaculate but who don't experience pleasurable sensations associated with it are sometimes described as having "ejaculatory anhedonia" or ejaculation without orgasm. Some men have always experienced ejaculation without any accompanying feelings of orgasm. Other men start out by having orgasmic ejaculations only to later notice a change in how it feels to ejaculate. Again, it's wise to see a health care provider to rule out medical conditions or medication side effects that may be causing this issue—especially if this is a sudden change that a man is experiencing. However, this issue is also often helped by seeing a sex therapist.

A Nose for Good Sex

Sex can be impacted by a number of factors, some of them quite unexpected. In a 2010 study published in the medical journal *The Laryngoscope,* medical researchers surgically treated patients with chronic sinusitis (a relatively common condition that causes a person's sinuses to become inflamed and swollen, which can lead to mucus buildup and difficulty breathing through one's nose).[9] Not only did the patients sleep better after treatment, but they also experienced improved sexual function. If you or your partner are suffering from a medical condition or an injury that gets in the way of sleep, it's probably getting in the way of sex too (lack of sleep does that, in addition to making people feel irritable and low on energy). Seek help from a health care provider for a chance at an overall better quality of life.

53. What to do if . . . he experiences painful ejaculation

Men who experience pain during ejaculation should let their health care provider know. Painful ejaculation is a rare problem, affecting about 1 to 5 percent of men. However, for those who experience ejaculatory pain, it's often a serious problem, as it can interfere with a man's relationships, love life, and sex life. Painful ejaculation is a rare side effect of some medications. The solution, therefore, may be as easy as stopping the medication under the advice or supervision of one's health care provider. However, there are a number of reasons why a man may experience pain during ejaculation, including prostate issues, obstruction of the ejaculatory ducts, and psychological issues. The first stop, then, is one's health care provider, such as a urologist, and the second stop (if still needed) is a sex therapist.

54. What to do if . . . he's bummed that his ejaculatory distance is down to inches rather than feet

Many men aren't told about the normal aspects of aging. If he was proud, in his twenties or thirties, about being able to shoot semen distances of several feet, he may feel disappointed that he no longer has the same "thrust" to his orgasms as he ages. Men can try to maintain muscle tone and thrust by doing Kegel exercises. Like women, they can do this by squeezing their pelvic floor muscles (the same ones that they can use to playfully make their penis "dance"), holding the contraction and then releasing it, repeating over and over again for several minutes per day. By exercising his pelvic floor muscles regularly, a man may be able to regain some ejaculatory distance. However, I know of no research on the topic, only anecdotal stories, so consider this a "can't hurt, might help" strategy. To a large extent, men, like women, often benefit from learning more about normal age-related changes. Some men feel reassured to know that there's not necessarily anything wrong with them or different about them for having less distance to their ejaculation than when they were younger. We're all aging—and our wonderful private parts age too, in their own way.

55. What to do if . . . he's got a case of the dribbles

Just as many men notice less distance to their ejaculation as they age, it is also common for men to experience less semen volume with age. Although it's not usually a noticeable decrease until later in years, scientific research has found that men's semen volume begins to decrease little by little in their twenties and keeps decreasing throughout life.

There has been strikingly little research on this phenomenon. In 2011, the topic came up on a sexual medicine–related email listserv that I am on and I was struck by the number of physicians who recommended that men who want to increase their semen volume do things like drink more water, eat certain foods, or take certain vitamins. In fact, I know of no research that suggests that drinking extra water or taking any of the vitamins actually works to help men produce more semen. I know of another man (who works in the porn industry) who firmly believes that eating celery is what helps him produce large amounts of semen. Again, though, I know of no scientific evidence to suggest that celery has anything to do with semen volume.

What we do know is this: men who smoke cigarettes tend to have less semen volume than men who don't smoke. Quitting smoking might help a man restore some of his lost semen volume or at least help slow down the rate of decrease. Also, men with larger waistlines are more likely to have less semen volume than thinner men. This may mean that adopting healthy lifestyle behaviors (like eating smaller portion sizes, choosing healthy foods, and exercising) may help men have or maintain more semen as well.

Sex Smarts Quiz

1. A man who frequently takes a very long time to ejaculate (often forty-five minutes or longer) may be said to have
    a. Delayed ejaculation
    b. Inhibited ejaculation
    c. Premature ejaculation
    d. Retrograde ejaculation
2. With age, men often experience _____ in the volume of semen that they produce.
    a. An increase
    b. A decrease
    c. No change
3. Researchers have found that all of the following can help to improve men's erectile and ejaculatory function except:
    a. Yoga
    b. Eating a Mediterranean diet
    c. Exercising
    d. All of the above have been shown to enhance men's sexual function

Answers
    1. a
    2. b
    3. d

Chapter 6
When Bodies Collide: The Good, the Bad, and the Sweaty Aspects of Partner Sex

When two people have sex, predictability can go right out the window. People have different wants and needs and different ideas about how often they should have sex—or certain types of sex—together. The partner you met isn't necessarily the same partner six months (or six years) later. Having a great sex life is, in large part, an experience in improv: you show up and roll with what life brings you, knowing that it can and will change each day. After all, nearly all couples will experience differences in sexual desires or preferred frequencies if they stay together long enough. It's how they manage these differences that makes for a delightful duo or a broken affair or marriage.

There are other predictably unpredictable aspects to sex too. Sex is full of various sights, sounds, scents, textures, not to mention fluids (yes, fluids). Then there are the emotions—yours and your partner's—that manifest themselves during sex in happy tears, frustrated tears, joyful giggles, shy gazes, and lustful looks.

But just because your sex life can't be perfectly predicted doesn't mean you can't prepare for it. In this chapter, we'll talk about common differences in desire, ways that women intuitively manage their own sexual desire and interest, attraction to one's partner, what happens when you desire someone who isn't your partner, and a hodgepodge of sex mishaps and concerns that leave many women wondering what to do (but not you; after reading this chapter *you'll know*).

WHAT MAKES FOR GOOD SEX?

Rarely is sex only about having babies. Even among couples who are trying to conceive, most times when they have sex there is low to no risk of pregnancy (unless they are undergoing serious fertility treatments that lead to frequent ovulation). Most of the time, women are not able to become pregnant because there's no egg sitting around waiting for a man's sperm to fertilize it. Women who have sex with women and men who have sex with men aren't able to have a baby from sex with their partner. And for postmenopausal women, sex is never again about having babies because the reproductive years are over.

This is important: it means that most of the sex human beings have, and will ever have, is not about making babies (the "work" of sex) but about sex for the sake of pleasure, connection, love, excitement, or whatever else it is that two people get from having sex with one another (the "playful side" of sex).

If sex is only sometimes about procreation and is mostly about recreation, then it's worth asking: What makes for good sex? Why is some sex so-so whereas other sexual experiences are nothing short of incredible? Why is one instance of sex boring and another exciting? How come some sexual experiences feel empty and others feel connecting and meaningful?

Scientists—like many women and men—have long pondered these questions. Much research has focused on sexual satisfaction and relationship satisfaction. Scientists who study sex have largely found that a person's sexual and relationship satisfaction are largely interconnected.[1-2] That is, when one is high, the other one is usually high too—and when one is low, the other one is usually also low. It's tough to tease out the differences between feeling satisfied sexually and satisfied in one's relationship and marriage. And yet there are couples for whom there is a clear distinction. I've talked with many women and men who say that they are happy with their relationship or marriage yet are sexually unsatisfied. They get along well with their partner, have pleasant dinners, pay the bills on time, have fun together at parties, are good parents to their kids, and so on. It's a "functional" relationship in the sense that it works. Yet sexually they may feel alone or unfulfilled, if they're even having sex at all. Some people can be great companions and friends to one another but get to a point where they feel more like roommates than people who want to get naked and roll around in a bed together. What, then, helps people have better sex?

A 2007 study published in the *Journal of Social and Personal Relationships* looked at the following characteristics and their importance to "good sex": competence, relatedness, and autonomy.[2] In my personal life, and when I teach about sex, I find these to be incredibly important components of "good sex" that aren't talked about enough.

Competence

People feel competent when they feel confident about doing the things they want to do. A major reason I wanted to write *Sex Made Easy* was so that more women could feel confident—and competent—about their sexual abilities. I want you to know that you can tackle almost any sexual situation you encounter. Feeling competent in your sex life can include feeling like you know how to use a sex toy to stimulate your body, perform oral sex on a partner, or ask for something sexual that you want. Some people come to feel sexually competent by noticing how their partner's body responds when they touch, lick, or stroke their partner—such as noticing that when they do these things their partner's penis gets hard or their partner's vagina gets wetter.

In pursuit of good sex, it's important to help your partner feel more competent too. When your partner does something that thrills you, speak up. Let your partner know when you've just enjoyed sex, when an orgasm has felt particularly good, or when you've especially enjoyed their oral sex technique or that thing they did with their hips, lips, or hands. Compliments and praise go a long way in the bedroom.

Relatedness

A sense of relatedness is about feeling connected to another person or having a feeling of belonging. It's about feeling like you understand your partner and that your partner understands or "sees" you for who you are. It's about intimacy and sharing yourself with another person, sexually as well as emotionally. You can meet your needs for relatedness (and thus increase your chances for feeling more sexually satisfied) by letting your partner know how you feel. Say things like "I really like you" or "I'm completely in love with you"—or however you feel comfortable expressing your feelings. You can further boost relatedness for yourself and your partner (thus increasing the likelihood that your partner will enjoy your sex life too) by finding more ways to connect. Ask your partner what he or she likes about your sex life. Ask what you do well or what turns them on. Share what turns you on. And if you find yourself in a place where you think to yourself, "I can't say that—he'll think I'm strange," that may be the very thing you need to share in order to cross the bridge and be truly intimate together. Being intimate with a person isn't limited to the mundane stuff of daily living, like how dark you like your toast or whether you sleep on the left or the right side of the bed. Being intimate involves courage and taking chances. You only earn the chance to feel like your partner "sees" you and gets you if you show yourself to your partner in the first place. People who hide their emotions and true selves from their partners don't stand much of a chance of feeling seen, heard, or understood. Don't be the person who hides. Be the partner who puts it out there and wants to be understood. Try your best to get to know your partner too, and to see past the everyday fronts and barriers people hide their true selves behind.

Autonomy

When it comes to sex, autonomy is about feeling like you're in charge of your sex life. You get to make choices about what you do sexually and whom you do it with. No one is making you do anything sexual or making you feel guilty if you don't want to have sex (guilt is one way of trying to make another person have sex). People who feel autonomous are people who feel that the things they do are things they *want* to do. This is one that I find very easy to relate to because it's been important to me my whole life, and not just in relation to sex. I can remember a time when I was a small child and was lying on my bed, pouting in my room. Just when I was thinking about leaving my bedroom and joining my family (who had friends visiting) in the living room, my mom came into the room. She told me that I needed to come and join everyone in the living room and that it would be a nice thing to do. Although she was well intentioned, her timing couldn't have been worse as far as I was concerned. I had been mentally preparing to come and join everyone—and it was all my idea, which made me feel good. Instead, she beat me to the punch, and now it would seem as if I were only leaving my room because she made me. Where was the pride or joy in that? I still feel this way as an adult in the sense that I am most proud of things I choose to do—and I feel less positively about things that other people have "suggested" I do (or tried to make me do). Can you think of examples in your own life where this has been the case?

In regard to sex, you may feel more sexually satisfied if you sometimes initiate sex rather than if your partner is always the one asking to have sex. If your partner is always asking, why not say to your partner something like, "I'd like to initiate sex more often. I know it might sound odd, but can you wait to initiate so that I get a turn to approach you for sex the next time? I want it to be my turn and my idea."

You might also be able to feel more autonomous by being the one who suggests using a vibrator or by saying you'd like to switch sex positions. If you feel that your partner pressures you into sex or tries to make you feel guilty about how often (or how seldom) you want sex, you may need to be assertive with your partner and ask them to lay off you. You may have different wants and needs from one another, which is common and healthy. Now you two need to find a way to both be satisfied with what you want—or, to want what you have.

Remember, too, that in order to feel sexually satisfied your partner may also need to feel autonomous about sex. If you're the one who's always initiating sex, try to give your partner space to initiate sometimes. Let him or her know that you'd love it, and feel more desirable, if they initiated sex more often—even if only once in a while. Make sure to listen to your partner when he or she shares something personal. By listening to your partner's sexual likes, dislikes, fantasies, or wants, you're showing your partner that you respect him or her as an autonomous individual, and that's important to both your experiences of sexual satisfaction.

If any one of these aspects of "good sex" resonates with you, consider reading *Passionate Marriage* by David Schnarch; it's one of my favorite books and I recommend it to couples who are looking to reignite passion, excitement, and closeness in their sexual and romantic relationships.

The Desire Dilemma

In our National Survey of Sexual Health and Behavior, we found that about 20 percent of women who didn't live with their partner—and about 25 percent of those who did—reported little or no sexual desire for their partner in the previous month (about half as many men in relationships reported little to no desire). Clearly, sexual desire presents a dilemma for many women and men. So what do they do about it? In another study, a colleague and I asked women about what's worked for them in times in which they or their partner have struggled with differences in desire. Their strategies included

- Scheduling sex
- Talking dirty
- Watching porn, together or alone
- Using sex toys
- Reading books about sex
- Going on romantic dates
- Wearing sexy clothes
- Using lubricant
- Marriage counseling, couples counseling, or sex therapy
- Sexual fantasy
- Cuddling
- Communicating more
- Agreeing on a frequency of sex that works for both partners
- Getting more sleep
- Having sex in places other than the bedroom
- Trying not to make a big deal out of whether or not sex happens
- Exercise and finding other ways to "de-stress"
- Massage and other forms of physical intimacy

• Talking about each other's insecurities and feelings

As of this writing, there are no FDA-approved medications to enhance women's or men's sexual desire (even if there were, they probably wouldn't work for everyone, as desire is impacted by so many things such as body image, relationship dynamics, health, and so on). There is no "quick fix" and no strategy that works for everyone; however, my hope is that this list gives you several ideas to try if you and your partner are working out desire differences of your own.

SEXUAL ATTRACTION

Of course, it would be naïve to think that sexual satisfaction is only about feeling connected, autonomous, and competent about sex. Clearly, feeling attracted to one's partner has to be somewhat important too, right? One would think so.

Yet this is an area of sexual satisfaction that has rarely been researched. Recently, I had the pleasure of working with a colleague (Kristen Mark) on a study about sexual desire, attraction, and sexual satisfaction among women who had been with their male partners for at least five years. We surveyed 176 women and asked them a number of questions about their partner and their relationship, including how attracted they felt to their partner and how this had changed over time (for example, whether they felt more or less attracted to him compared to when they first met, or if their attraction to him was about the same).[4] We found that for this group of women, their current attraction to their partner and their change in attraction over time were better predictors of their sexual satisfaction than were their levels of relationship satisfaction. This supports the idea that in order to be sexually satisfied in one's relationship it isn't always enough to work well together and do things like take out the garbage or talk about each other's days (the whole "functional relationship" idea). These are important parts of living well together and loving one another, but there's more to feeling happy with one's sex life than the day-to-day aspects of living together. Feeling attracted to each other matters too.

This is also backed up by something I regularly hear from men and women, which is the issue of feeling less attracted to one's partner who has "let themselves go." It seems that this phrase was long applied mostly to women—the stereotypical idea being that once a woman got married, she stopped trying to look good and let her looks fall by the wayside. However, men aren't the only ones who value physical attractiveness, and I just as often hear women complain that their (male or female) partners don't pay enough attention to their appearance. This seems to have intensified for men as more pressure has been placed on them to adopt "metrosexual" behaviors such as dressing more fashionably, grooming their eyebrows, and even grooming their pubic hair.

Of course, beauty truly is in the eye of the beholder and people are attracted to individuals with a wide range of body types, hair colors, skin colors, hair styles, ethnicities, and heights. However, there's no denying that people like what they like, and while they can often learn to appreciate a person who looks different from what they find attractive, they may never have the same gut reaction of pure physical attraction to somebody who doesn't fall at least loosely within their personal perceptions of what it means to be "attractive."

A few examples from my work life come to mind. One is a letter I once received from a man whose wife had gained a significant amount of weight in the first year they were married (something like thirty or forty pounds). I say this is "significant" because thirty or forty pounds is a lot of weight to gain—or lose—in the span of one year. This man wrote to me because he was feeling terrible. He wanted to have more frequent sex, yet he was no longer sexually attracted to his wife and had tried to encourage her to lose weight so that he would find her physically attractive again. She responded with something along the lines of "If you loved me, my weight wouldn't matter." He insisted that he still loved her—but that he wasn't nearly as attracted to her as he once was. (Ouch.)

Now, I happen to love and be fascinated by the range of body shapes that exist in the world, and I think we could all use a lot less stigma and busy-body-ness about each other's weight, size, and shape. However, I also agree that love and attraction are often two very different experiences. While love and attraction often go together, it isn't always the case. If the man who wrote to me was attracted to women in a certain range of body weight, then a thirty- or forty-pound weight gain (or loss) could have considerably changed the way his wife looked (and I have no idea what body weight she started out with, whether she was very skinny, average, or of a larger size) and thus significantly changed his attraction to her. Is that fair? No. Is it a reality for some women and men? Yes. These days it's not politically correct for people to talk openly about losing attraction to someone when they gain or lose weight; however, it's a reality that many people experience.

Several women in their fifties once told me similar stories about their husbands. Of the group of women, only one of them worked full time outside the home. Mostly, they were busy raising their children and managing their households, and all of them prioritized working out and eating healthy meals. Their husbands, on the other hand, were successful businessmen who traveled frequently for work. Each of these women was strong, fit, thin or of average body weight, and an avid exerciser. All but one complained that their husbands had gained a lot of weight since their marriages, and all but one said that they found this unattractive and something that had negatively influenced their sexual desire for their husbands. These women all described feeling very much in love with their husbands and committed to their marriages; but they also said that they were no longer attracted to their husbands because of their weight and had sex largely out of obligation ("duty sex") and not from desire or attraction. There was a great deal of sadness in these women's stories as they struggled to make sense of the disconnect between their feelings of love and lack of attraction for their husbands. Given the sensitivity of talking about weight issues, not one of them had felt comfortable enough to broach the issue with their husbands or to be honest about their lack of desire.

Politically correct or not, this happens: many people find that their sexual attraction (and related desire and sexual satisfaction) is influenced by their partner's appearance—and, I would add, probably by society's often judgmental attitudes about appearance. On the other end of the weight spectrum, a number of the male college students I teach have talked with me about losing attraction to their girlfriends who starve themselves to the point of being very skinny. "I liked how soft she used to feel," I remember one guy saying. "Now she's all bony and pointy and obsessed with being skinny." Also, it's not only weight that can influence sexual attraction: hair length and color can influence sexual attraction; body composition (being softer versus more muscular); height; how white or straight one's teeth are; and so on.

It's not even always how a person's *partner* looks that matters. Research has found that how women and men feel about their *own bodies,* and their own looks, is important to how they feel sexually, especially in older age. And although research has focused mainly on women's body image in older age, many men feel similarly challenged by body image concerns. A number of research studies have shown that it's not body size, but body image, that's most relevant to people's sexual lives.[5-6] Women and men of all shapes and sizes can have active, healthy, enjoyable, exciting, and highly sexy sex lives; sex is definitely not only for the skinny, despite what you may see on television, in the movies, in mainstream porn, or represented in lingerie catalogs. Sex is for all of us—and it can be enjoyed by all of us—particularly when we feel confident and positive about our bodies (this includes our butts, thighs, stomachs, arms, breasts, genitals, faces, and everything else).

Women and, increasingly men, also worry about growing less attractive to their partner as they grow older. Having grown up in Miami, Florida—a city with more than its fair share of people obsessed with plastic surgery and looking younger—I am all too familiar with watching husbands and wives trade in their spouses for a "younger model." Two that come immediately to mind are a mid-forties businessman who left his same-aged wife for the secretary half his age, and the early-forties stay-at-home mom who left her slightly older CEO husband for her much younger yoga instructor.

So how do we manage attraction? And how do we keep ourselves attractive to our partner (and attractive to ourselves)? Some of it has to do with adopting healthy lifestyle behaviors: eating well, exercising, and so on. For many people, when they look good, they feel good. The key word, however, is "healthy." Because being overweight and looking old are so terribly stigmatized in many cultures, people often try anything to lose weight or look younger (including risky cosmetic surgeries) in order to reach these goals. If you would like to adopt different eating or exercise behaviors, I recommend checking in with a health care provider and a registered dietician to learn more about healthy eating and exercise.

Some of it also has to do with our perspectives and our communication with our partners. For this reason, I also recommend talking with your partner. Oftentimes we think our partner wants us to look like something we're not—and often we're wrong about what they find attractive. As an example, if your partner watches porn that features skinny women with breast implants, it doesn't necessarily mean that that's what he or she finds attractive, or that your partner finds you unattractive if your body is shaped differently from those women's bodies. Raising the issue with your partner may help provide you with more information about what he or she finds attractive. It may also give you an opportunity to share what you find attractive about your partner—and about your own body. You may find that your bedmate doesn't want you to change a thing about yourself, and he or she might find it sexy to hear how much you love your curves, breasts, hips, freckles, tan lines, nose, pale skin, or whatever else you enjoy about your body. All too often we share what we're dissatisfied about in terms of our bodies. But it could do us all some good to share with one another what we like about ourselves and our bodies, what turns us on, and what we hope will turn our partner on as well. Try it and see for yourself. Try to identify what you love about your body and share that with your partner. Let your partner know what you like about their body too. Compliment your partner on their butt, on how they look in their jeans, or on how it feels when they wrap their arms around you (loving a person's body isn't always about how it looks, but how it feels, too).

There's another reason to talk openly with your partner about your feelings of attraction. Remember the concept of "relatedness"? If we hide our feelings from our partner, we don't get the chance to feel understood—or to reach out and understand them. Three times in my life I fell hard in love (and lust) for men whose body types were different from the body types I typically find attractive. Two of these men are individuals with whom I experienced far greater than average intimacy and emotional closeness. It may be that even if your partner's body or other parts of their appearance are different from your "type," a sense of relatedness and intimacy will bridge those differences, which may not ultimately matter at all.

To be interested in the changing seasons is a happier state of mind than to be hopelessly in love with spring.
—George Santayana

SELF-EXPANSION: WHEN YOU AND I BECOME "US"

There's another aspect to feeling satisfied in a relationship and feeling attracted and "into" another person, and this is something called "self-expansion."[7-8] Some of my favorite research about relationships has examined love from this perspective. The idea is that people often look for romantic and sexual relationships that make them feel bigger than they are all by themselves.

Think about your own life for a moment and think specifically about people you have dated, been romantically or sexually involved with, or have had a serious crush on. Chances are, you felt like some of these people expanded your world by introducing you to new people, music, hobbies, interests, food, sports, and so on.

When I think back on my own life and relationships, I can say this: although I've had the pleasure of participating in several sprint triathlons, I signed up for my first one because a guy I liked was into sprint triathlons and his stories about them fascinated me. And as for music, a look through the music folder on my laptop is like peeking into my past relationships. It's filled with songs that I know and love because people I once dated, or had crushes on, put the songs on mix tapes or emailed them to me. Others are songs I became familiar with because an ex and I would sit around the house and he would excitedly say "you've got to listen to this song." He would play it, and I would learn it, and the world as I knew it got bigger and bigger— and with a much better soundtrack than I could manage on my own.

We tend to like people who expose us to new things, who introduce us to something about the world that we didn't see or notice or appreciate before. I've introduced exes to yoga, gardening, folk music, indie bands, cooking, hiking, vegetarian restaurants, travel, and occasionally sex toys and the Stop-Start Technique detailed in chapter 5 (we all have our own special things to offer). What have you introduced your present or former partners to?

We tend to be less into people who don't expand our world, who don't show us anything new or interesting. To the extent you can, then, try to show your partner more about who you are and what you have to offer. You're not responsible for everything about your relationship; your partner has to be open to seeing you in all your glory and learning from you, just as you need to be open to learning something new from your partner. I often tell people that when they think they know everything there is to know or see about their partner, that is when they can probably say with confidence that they're wrong. If you want to stay together, don't give up on learning new aspects of your partner. Keep looking. Keep asking questions. Keep sharing new things about yourself, and maybe your partner will open up bit by bit as well. Self-expansion isn't only about learning new songs or recipes; it's about being more intimate with each other and building your sense of relatedness (there we go again).

WHEN SOMEONE ELSE STARTS TO LOOK GOOD

Now it's time to talk about a topic that I find is rarely openly discussed: the experience of being attracted to, or developing a crush on, someone other than the person you're in a relationship with. While it's somewhat expected that people who are casually dating are checking out and comparing their options (mentally assessing whether the person they're dating is a better or worse potential mate than their cute coworker), an awful lot of silence falls around this topic for people who are in serious relationships or who are married. But being in love and committed to a partner, or married to them, doesn't preclude having feelings for other people.

This isn't even necessarily about cheating. It's about taking an honest appraisal of the experience of being human. Living with someone or wearing a ring around your finger doesn't mean that you stop noticing other people. Sure, some people do. But most women and men that I hear from in my research and in my classes will describe having been attracted to, or romantically interested in, someone other than their partner; they just don't often talk about it openly for fear that they will be judged or that their partner will feel insecure or threatened or worry that they will cheat. Then again, some people have relationships in which they and their partners can openly and honestly talk about having crushes on other people or fantasizing about what it would be like to have sex with someone else. And some people have open relationships in which they can and do have sex with others.

In one research study, a colleague and I asked women who had been in long-term relationships whether or not they had had a crush on someone other than their partner, or if they'd been sexually attracted to someone else such as a friend, former partner, coworker, or even a celebrity. Many women shared their stories with us. Among their stories were Facebook flirtations, coworkers they wondered about, attractive people they noticed in passing, friends, and exes.

Some of these experiences are ones that the women in our study seemed to identify as fleeting and not necessarily as threats to their relationship. One woman, for example, wrote,

> *Every few years or so, I have had a crush on someone or other, a friend, an employee, a celebrity, or an old boyfriend. These take the form of a mental fantasy or obsession for several days or a few weeks. I get turned on imagining a fling and a period of sexual discovery, and then it passes.*

Although many women kept their attractions secret and didn't mention anything to their partner, some women wrote about being able to talk openly with their partner about their attractions:

> *I shared with my husband that I have always been attracted to women. I have never acted on this while we have been married, but now I can talk about it. I have never desired to be with another man other than my husband, however.*

Several women, including this one, wrote about attractions that were based on online interactions with offline implications:

> *Facebook has reconnected me to past boyfriends. I have had dreams involving people I have slept with in the past.*

There are also, of course, women who experience their attractions as something they might take a step further. Some women wrote about realizing that they wanted to have sex with another person, or that they might be vulnerable to cheating on their partner if they let themselves be alone with the person they felt attracted to or had a crush on. Others seemed to be actively considering opportunities to have sex with someone else, such as this woman who wrote,

> *Cuz I don't have sex with my hubby, I always am thinking about cheating on him. He doesn't like sex or want it. I have not cheated on him yet but I am thinking about it. If I felt safe with other men and could trust them, I would do it. Whenever I see some cute guy I think I should have sex with him, especially in the gym.*

And in some cases, women wrote about the damage caused by their attractions and by their actual affairs:

> *I discovered I had attractions for other people a few years into my marriage. It created a rift in our relationship until I was able to be completely open and honest with my partner.*

> *I fell in love with someone else once, and it was a very painful experience. It wasn't just sexual, but emotional and mental as well. However, I made the choice to end this affair, though every now and then I still think about him.*

However, not all of the "explored attractions" that have resulted in sex with another person have been damaging. For some women, experiencing attraction to another person led them to reconsider what they wanted and to talk about it with a partner. One woman wrote,

> *I have had a series of attractions for others throughout our relationship. About one and a half years ago I began an experience of very strong attraction for a person and that is what eventually brought me to bring up the possibility of an open relationship with my husband, so I could explore a relationship with the other person. As he also had experienced attractions for others, he was interested and we proceeded to open things up.*

There are no hard and fast rules about feeling attracted to, or sexually or romantically interested in, someone other than your partner—and there is very little scientific research on the topic outside of all-out affairs. If you find yourself crushing on or fantasizing about someone else, you may find it helpful to know how other women manage their feelings so you can sort out the best path for yourself. Aside from having an affair, some women manage their crushes by:

- Trying to distance themselves from their crush
- Making sure they aren't alone with the other person
- Making sure they aren't drunk around the other person
- Not giving it a second thought, with the expectation that the feelings will pass
- Masturbating
- Fantasizing about the other person, but with the knowledge that it's only a fantasy and nothing they are pursuing in real life
- If the crush is someone they used to date, reminding themselves that they broke up for a reason
- Having frequent sex with their partner so they don't feel extra desire for the other person
- Writing a letter to the person and then throwing it away
- Being open and honest with their partner about the feelings
- Talking with their partner about opening up their relationship

Having a crush on another person is a common, human experience—even when you are madly in love with your partner. It doesn't mean you're a bad person or that your relationship is doomed. However, it may not be an "easy" experience for you to deal with depending on the depth of your feelings for this other person. Hopefully, hearing other women's stories and thinking about the many options available to you will be helpful as you work to figure out the best path for you and your partner.

— Making It Easy —

56. What to do if . . .you can't "feel anything" during sex

This typically isn't about anything "wrong" with your body. Rather, you may simply be very aroused and thus producing lots of vaginal lubrication that has decreased friction and thus decreased sensation. Or, if you've added store-bought lubricant to the mix, perhaps you've added too much. No worries: grab a soft towel or use the sheets and dab your genitals, and possibly your partner's genitals, and then resume sex. It should feel tighter and like you can "feel" more. If there are no sheets or towels nearby and your partner is a man, you can sometimes use your hand to rub his penis up and down (like you're giving him a hand job) as a way to dry his genitals (any wetness from your vagina that was left on his penis will come off on your hands and mostly absorb into your skin). Again, sex should feel more sensation packed post–dry off.

This assumes, of course, that your male partner has an erect penis that is somewhere in the average or above average range. If his penis, even when erect, is quite small (say, in the one- to three-inch range) and thin, then you may not be feeling much because, well, there's not a whole lot to feel unless you have an extra small-sized vagina yourself ; see chapter 2 for more on sex with a man whose penis is on the small side.

If you never feel much during sex, mention this to your gynecologist or whichever health care provider does your GYN exams. Sometimes women who experience vaginal wall relaxation (often marked by genital prolapse) feel as though they've lost vaginal sensation during sex and don't feel much. Depending on how severe the prolapse is, your health care provider may even recommend a surgical procedure that can improve any continence issues you may be experiencing (for example, peeing when you don't mean to pee or passing frequent or excessive gas). Sexual function, including vaginal sensation during sex, also often improves following these front-wall and back-wall repair surgeries for prolapse.

You may see creams or gels for sale that are marketed as vaginal "tighteners" or that promise to make you feel almost "virginal" again (referring to vaginal tightness). These often contain an ingredient that causes vaginal inflammation and/or dryness, which is why sex may feel tighter afterwards. I am not personally a fan of these substances because I generally feel protective of women's vaginas and the things that happen to them. However, I understand that there are many women who lack sensation during sex (for reasons related to prolapse or having a small-sized partner, for example) and who may choose to use such creams or gels. I support women's rights to make their own choices about their bodies—but I do want you to understand what these creams and gels do to the body so that you can feel more informed about your options.

57. What to do if . . . you run out of lube in the midst of sex, and need more

Easy: if you're using water-based lubricant, dip your fingers into a nearby cup or bowl of room-temperature water that you've laid out ahead of time on your bedside nightstand and use it to rewet your or your partner's genitals. Water-based lube often absorbs into the skin but can be reawakened with a little water. Or you can simply add more water-based lubricant. It doesn't last very long, which isn't a big deal for most people's sex lives. However, some people spend a considerable amount of time in sex and may benefit from adding more lubricant from time to time for more comfortable, pleasurable, low-friction sex.

If you're not into the idea of having to frequently reapply lubricant, then the next time you anticipate spending a long time having sex, choose a silicone-based lubricant. Silicone-based lube lasts longer during sex. That said, it shouldn't be used with silicone-based products such as silicone-based contraceptives (like cervical caps) or silicone sex toys.

58. What to do if . . . your libidos don't match

Join the club. If you stay with a partner long enough and make a relationship out of it, there are likely to be times in your lives when your libidos—or sexual preferences—don't exactly match up. Your partner might want sex once a week and you might long for it every day (or vice versa). Some people can go stretches of time without sex and others want it more often. Then there are all the other ways people sometimes want different things; for example, one person wants sex at night before going to sleep but their partner, who's more of a morning person, would rather do it first thing after waking up.

If you're mismatched in this way, it's not necessarily cause for alarm. You can work this out. If there's a significant gap in your sexual desires, you may want to ask yourselves whether you're both content to be monogamous or if you want to open your relationship in some way so that one or both of you is "allowed" to kiss other people or engage in some type of sex (e.g., oral sex, vaginal sex, anal sex) with other people. There is very little research on open relationships and we don't know how common, or rare, they are, though they seem to be more common among gay male couples than heterosexual or lesbian couples (likely because, generally speaking, men tend to have higher sex drives and more permissive attitudes about sex). However, opening one's relationship—whether a little bit or a lot—is one way some couples manage mismatched libidos.

If you decide to stay monogamous (which many people do as well), you need to figure out a way to manage your libidos so that both partners feel like they won. If all you do is meet in the middle, both partners may feel as though they've lost a little. You might ask yourselves: Can the person who wants sex more often be content to make up for the difference with masturbation? Is the person who wants sex less often willing to, and interested in, making up the difference with oral sex, mutual masturbation, hand jobs, sex toy play, or heated makeout sessions? Does the person who wants sex less often have needs that are going unmet? Would he or she want sex more often if only there were more emotional intimacy, or a willingness to try new sexual things, or if their partner helped out around the house more? Thinking about these issues can help you and your partner figure out what you can do to change your sex life for the better without pressuring one another to be something they're not.

59. What to do if . . . you're in a sexless relationship— and want the sex to come back!

If you and your partner aren't having sex and you're unhappy about this, you absolutely must talk to your partner about it. If your partner is happy not having sex and you're not, ask your partner if he or she is willing to see a sex therapist together with you. Even if his or her goal isn't to ever have sex with you again, it's worth trying to see if there is some way you can reconnect or even restructure your relationship.

For example, some couples agree that it is unlikely they will ever have sex again but decide to stay together because they love each other, want to be together, and want, perhaps, to continue raising their children together. If one person has completely lost interest in having sex, however, that person sometimes gives their partner the green light to seek sex elsewhere. This doesn't work for all couples but it is one way some couples manage this difference and stay together. Other times, if one person has decided they're not interested in sex at all—and the other feels sex is important to them—they decide to part ways and separate or divorce. I recommend meeting with a sex therapist and/or couples therapist before separating, as often a relationship/marriage can indeed be saved.

On the other hand, if your partner wants to have sex again too—and you just aren't sure where to begin—simply go for it. Try and try again. Commit to each other that you will try, even if the sex is awkward and fumbling at first. You are in this together and want to be back to wherever you were before in your sex lives (you know, when you used to have sex). You might try having sex together after sharing a bottle of wine. Or sign up for a weekend sex therapy workshop retreat together. You might even start seeing a sex therapist on a regular basis. If you're open to reading a book on the topic, check out *Passionate Marriage* by Dr. David Schnarch, one of my favorite books for rekindling passion within long-term relationships. If you and your partner worry that you are a lost cause, let me reassure you: I know of couples who have gone fifteen years or more without having sex even once and they have been helped by a good sex therapist. It is absolutely possible to get your sex life back whether it's been eight months, two years (and two kids), or fifteen years or longer. Go for it.

60. What to do if . . . you feel pressured to have sex or guilted into it

An occasional instance of "duty sex" isn't so bad. In fact, a number of women and men sometimes have sex when they don't feel like it for the simple reason that their partner feels like having sex and they want to do something nice for their partner. Plus—as an added bonus—sometimes people get into sex once they start kissing and hugging and touching and then start thinking, "This is fun! I'm glad I went for this." Win-win.

There's a difference between sensing your partner wants to do it and saying "sure" and feeling pressured or guilted into sex you don't want. If you feel like your partner is pressuring you to have sex when you've made it clear that you don't want to, call him or her on it. Say something like, "I'm feeling pressured to have sex with you right now, which I don't like. Let's take a step back for a minute" or "I'm sure you're not trying to make me feel bad for not wanting to have sex right now, but it feels that way."

If you notice that you're frequently not feeling into sex, don't gloss over what could become an issue for your relationship. Ask yourself what's going on and what your reasons are for not wanting to be sexual with your partner. Are you feeling tired? Misunderstood? Overworked or ignored? As if your partner doesn't "see you" or "get you"? Talk with your partner about whatever it is you're going through so that he or she doesn't feel flat-out rejected, unloved, or unattractive as a result of you not feeling in the mood for sex. Read more detailed how-to suggestions and exercises for learning to say yes to sex you do want and no to sex you don't in *Because It Feels Good: A Woman's Guide to Sexual Pleasure and Satisfaction*.

61. What to do if . . . you can't use hormonal birth control but don't want to get pregnant yet

Easy! Modern technology has given you multiple options for nonhormonal birth control. Condoms are a great birth control option. They're affordable, and, as long as you're not allergic to the materials they're made with, there are no side effects to condom use. Condoms are also a wise option for people who are even slightly concerned about STI risk, such as if your partner has an STI (such as herpes or HPV) and you want to do whatever you can to reduce your risk of getting it—even if you know condoms can't provide 100 percent protection. It's also smart to use condoms with a partner if there's a chance that you or he/she might have sex with someone else, like if you're in that hazy phase of not being entirely certain how trustworthy your partner is or whether you're totally exclusive with one another.

If you're not worried about STI risk (for example, if you and your partner have been tested for STIs together and are comfortable with each other's STI status), you can use the withdrawal (pulling-out) method, which can work well as long as your partner is super good about pulling his penis out of your vagina before even a drop of semen spurts out of his penis. If he's not so good at that, why not use condoms plus withdrawal, thus increasing the odds that you two will be well protected from pregnancy?

There are other birth control options available for women and men who aren't worried about STI risk and who don't want to use a hormonal method of birth control. Ask your health care provider for more information about the cervical cap, a barrier device that's fitted over the cervix to keep sperm from swimming through the cervix and into the uterus and fallopian tubes to find a waiting egg. You can also talk to your health care provider about intrauterine devices (IUD). IUDs are put into place by a woman's health care provider and offer long-term birth control.

62. What to do if . . . your partner's oral skills are lacking

It happens. Sometimes, no matter how well two people communicate, one of them can't seem to put what they're hearing into practice. Your partner may be very clear that you prefer light tongue flicks that continue, uninterrupted, at a fast pace. However, maybe he's prone to a sore jaw. Or maybe he gets bored and is more turned on by long, slow licking of your vulva. Who knows? The point is that some folks don't do what one hopes, sexually speaking.

There's no real "easy" solution to this one. You can try—once again—to teach your partner what you like. If you go this route, try to compliment them on something they do well (Maybe they're a good kisser? Or they have a great way of stimulating your G Spot during vaginal sex?). After you've offered up a compliment, try saying something like "I think I would really be turned on by a little tweak to our oral sex play. Do you think you might try . . ." and then say what it is you're hoping that he or she will do. It may take demonstrating your licking or kissing or nibbling technique on his hand. You may find it helpful to practice a few times for the sake of fun, without any intention of it being a "real" sex session that results in an orgasm. Sometimes it's a good idea to simply explore sexually and learn what each other likes.

The challenge (and why this is not exactly an "easy" solution) is that your partner may feel offended. Their feathers may be ruffled over the idea that they're not giving you the amazing oral sex they thought they were giving. And if that's the case, there's not a lot you can do about it. This is a good reason why it's sometimes helpful to have these kinds of sex talks sometime when you are not about to have sex, in the midst of sex, or have just finished sex. Try talking about your sex life sometime when you're away from the bedroom and sitting around chatting, eating, or hanging out. Too few people talk about sex openly with their partner and it can do a world of good to try it.

Finally, you may have to face the fact that your partner cannot deliver the exact technique you want. That's humanity for you! We're all people and none of us is perfect. Try to widen the scope to include a range of sex acts that have major pleasure potential. It's not fair to insist that your partner has to get this one thing right when there are many other things that they could be doing well.

63. What to do if . . . you have a pregnancy scare

If you've somehow had unprotected sex—maybe because it was the heat of the moment and you forgot, or maybe because a condom broke or you realized too late that you had missed a few of your birth control pills—you may be able to take emergency contraception (EC), also known as the "morning-after pill." EC is most effective when taken within three days, or seventy-two hours, of unprotected sex. Note: if a woman is already pregnant, EC will not end or terminate the pregnancy—it is not an "abortion pill"; rather, EC can only reduce the likelihood of pregnancy occurring by preventing a woman from ovulating and making it more difficult for a fertilized egg to implant itself into the uterus.

If it's likely that you're pregnant, you may want to explore your options, which include terminating the pregnancy (abortion—call local clinics to learn more about this), adoption, and raising the baby. If you choose to continue with your pregnancy (whether you ultimately put your baby up for adoption or raise him or her), it's a very good idea to start prenatal health care as soon as you realize that you are pregnant. Your health care provider can talk with you about healthy pregnancy, including what you need to know about nutrition, exercise, abstaining from alcohol, quitting smoking, health care visits, and caring for your own health and that of your growing baby.

If it turns out that you are not pregnant, you might want to reassess how you feel. If you and your partner are not ready to become parents and feel relieved that you are not actually pregnant, you may want to look into using effective methods of birth control (visit www.plannedparenthood.org for information about contraceptive methods such as the birth control pill, patch, shot, and ring). If you are sort of sad or disappointed that you are not pregnant, you may want to ask yourself if you're in a different place in life than you perhaps realized. If you think you might be ready to become pregnant, talk with your partner about this possibility, as well as your health care provider, so that you can aim toward a healthy future pregnancy.

64. What to do if . . . your partner tries to have sex with you while they are sleeping

Urge your partner to see a sleep specialist. Many people who act out sexually during their sleep (such as masturbating oneself or trying to have sex with another person, and then not remembering any of it the next day) have a sleep disorder that is causing or contributing to this behavior. This is sometimes referred to as "sexsomnia."[9]

It's important to be checked out by a health care provider for several reasons. For one, your partner may not even realize they have poor sleep quality. They may often feel tired, irritable, or grumpy and not know why. If it turns out that they have a sleep disorder that can be treated, then better sleep for everyone may be just around the corner; the middle-of-the-night sexual advances might disappear too, helping you get sounder sleep as well. Another reason to seek treatment is that acting out sexually during sleep can challenge some relationships. You may feel scared or angry to wake up one night and find your partner on top of you attempting sex. Another risk is that, if left untreated, some people have been known to attempt to have sex, or to forcibly have sex, with others as part of their "sexsomnia" episodes. So even if it doesn't bother you or your partner, it may be a good idea to mention it to a health care provider.

Sex Smarts Quiz

1. Emergency contraception is most effective when taken
    a. Within three days of unprotected sex
    b. Within five days of unprotected sex
    c. Within a week of unprotected sex
    d. Any time at all
2. If you can't or don't want to use hormonal methods of birth control, other options include
    a. Condoms
    b. A nonhormonal IUD
    c. Withdrawal
    d. All of the above
3. Three important components of "good sex" are competence, autonomy, and
    a. Relationships
    b. Relatedness
    c. Reinforcement
    d. Regularity

Answers
    1. a
    2. d
    3. b

Chapter 7
Easy Does It:
Sex Toys, Joys, and Mishaps

Over the past decade, sex toys such as vibrators, dildos, and penis rings (also called c-rings, cock rings, and condom rings) have become very mainstream. Sex toys are no longer the purview of dimly lit adult bookstores frequented only by men. They can now be found in drugstores, women's in-home parties, high-end sex boutiques, medical offices, and on websites. As you'll see throughout this chapter, though, it hasn't always been an easy ride.

As the sex toy industry has expanded over the past decade, an increasing number of people are left with questions about how to use sex toys, how not to use them, what's risky, what's pleasurable, and what to do when things don't go as planned. A quick Internet search often yields conflicting information, leaving people even more uncertain about how to safely and pleasurably make sex toys a healthy part of their sexual lives. At conferences I attend, medical doctors and nurses talk about their struggles to stay up to date on issues related to sex toy use and lubricants so that they can better educate their patients and help them stay healthy (as you'll see later in this chapter, some people do some unusual and even dangerous things as part of their sex play).

Here you will find information about sex toys that you can trust, including a brief tutorial on sex toy materials, how to clean sex toys, and how to use different types of vibrators on your own body or a partner's body. By being more knowledgeable about sex toys, you will be able to feel more relaxed and confident using them and creating the pleasure that you deserve.

WHO USES VIBRATORS, ANYWAY?

In a 2009 issue of the *Journal of Sexual Medicine,* our Indiana University research team published data from the first-ever national probability study of vibrator use in the US, in which we found that vibrator use was far more common than many people previously knew. Far from being something unusual, a full 53 percent of women and nearly half of men ages eighteen to sixty in the US reported having used vibrators.[1-2] In addition, findings from our study demonstrated that vibrator use is linked to positive sexual function for women (for example, higher arousal, higher desire, less pain during sex, easier orgasm) as well as for men.

Most women in our study who used vibrators said that they had done so during masturbation as well as with a partner. Most of men's vibrator use was with a female sex partner such as a girlfriend or wife. That's not to say, though, that men never play with vibrators when they're on their own. We found that nearly one in five American men reported having used a vibrator during masturbation. This didn't entirely surprise me, as I've long received emails and letters from men who say that they sometimes explore with their girlfriend or wife's vibrator while she is out (this is one reason why it's wise to clean one's vibrator before each use!).

SECRET SEX TOYS

Of course, you don't have to take my word for it that vibrators and other sex toys have become common or mainstream. The next time you're shopping a local drugstore or retail chain store such as Duane Reade, CVS, Walmart, or Target, look around. There's a good chance that somewhere in the aisles you'll find a vibrator for sale. Although such stores may not sell the full range of vibrators that are commonly available in adult bookstores and sex boutiques (for example, the Silver Bullets and Rabbits of the world), vibrators sold in drugstores and mainstream retail stores can still be used to enhance masturbation and partner play quite pleasurably. For decades, mainstream stores have sold a number of what I call "secret sex toys": products that aren't necessarily sold as sex toys but are often used that way. Chief among these are vibrating "back massagers"— and while many people who buy these products truly do use them to massage their backs, a number of people use vibrating back massagers to stimulate their genitals.

How do I know? For starters, the Hitachi Magic Wand (a popular back massager) has been recommended for decades by artist, activist, and masturbation workshop leader Betty Dodson, something she writes about in her book *Sex for One*.[3] This particular back massager/vibrator is also on display in her video, *Selfloving*, which is about female masturbation and sexuality. And in *Becoming Orgasmic*, sex therapists Drs. Julia Heiman and Joseph LoPiccolo reference the use of back massagers for genital stimulation,[4] as does Rachel Maines in her book *The Technology of Orgasm*. But back massagers aren't the only secret sex toys or vibrating devices you'll find in a drugstore. You'll also find vibrating tooth brushes, which former students and readers of my sex columns have told me they've used as part of masturbation and sex play. Their vibrating intensity is on the lower end, but a number of people enjoy using them for sex play nevertheless (hopefully it goes without saying that you should not brush your or anyone else's teeth with a vibrating tooth brush that has been used on the genitals). Several column readers and students have also told me that they've used the nonrazor end of vibrating razors to stimulate their genitals. Clearly, one should always be careful when sharp objects go near one's genitals, but if you can play safely and carefully—such as while shaving your own or your partner's pubic hair—then have at it.

And in recent years, a number of mainstream stores have started selling vibrating condom rings, typically in the condom aisle. These vibrating rings are usually sold as single-use (disposable) flexible rings that are worn around a man's penis and that vibrate, stimulating his and his partner's genitals during partnered sex. Although they may be sold as "condom rings," one doesn't necessarily need to use the condom with the ring— though certainly safer sex is always a good idea.

Vibrators and other sex toys are also sold to literally millions of women each year through in-home sex toy parties. Some women feel more comfortable shopping for sex toys this way. In addition to serving as a fun "girls' night" among friends, for some women these parties feel more private and confidential than shopping for sex toys in a public setting such as a store. Some medical practices now sell vibrators and lubricants as well, particularly as more women and men seek help for sexual health issues from their doctor or nurse. Everyone has their own comfort zones, and the fact that sex toys are available through so many different venues means that most people who are interested in sex toys can probably find a way to get their hands on one.

WHY USE SEX TOYS?

Most people who bring sex toys into their masturbation or partnered sex play don't do so because they need to, but because they want to. In our 2009 study of vibrator use, we found that 58 percent of women who used vibrators said they started doing so for fun and 55 percent said it was out of curiosity. About a third of women said they started using vibrators to spice up their sex life or to make it easier for them to have an orgasm. And about a quarter said that they didn't have a sexual partner at the time and another 27 percent said they started using vibrators because their partner wanted to. These are all common and valid reasons why women (and men too) start to use vibrators. And while many people associate vibrator use with masturbation, it's also true that a person's partner sometimes influences their decision to give vibrator play a try. After all, a fun part of being sexual with another person is learning from them and trying new things together. All it takes sometimes is for one person to say to another, "I wonder what you'd think about . . ." and then suggesting something new, whether it's experimenting with using a vibrator, going to a sex club, kissing for hours, or having sex on the living room floor instead of retreating to the bedroom. In the case of sex toys, you can include your partner by shopping together for one online or in a local store, or showing them how your use your favorite toy during masturbation.

MAKING SEX BETTER

Of course, vibrators aren't the only sex toy. And while there's no agreed-upon definition for sexual enhancement product, I tend to think of it as an umbrella term for products that can make sex feel better for people. Sex toys are commonly considered to be sexual enhancement products, as they're generally marketed as products meant to make sex more fun, novel, or potentially more easily orgasmic. Sex toys include vibrators, dildos, penis rings, and a whole range of other sex toys such as butt plugs, nipple clamps, handcuffs, feathers, whips, body frosting, edible body powder, and more.

I consider lubricants to be a type of sexual enhancement product too, because they can also make masturbation and partnered sex better for people and are often marketed in this manner. In one national study, we found that 62 percent of women had ever used a vibrator.[5] In another scientific study conducted by my Indiana University research team, we gave more than twenty-four hundred women one of six different water-based or silicone-based lubricants as part of one of the world's largest studies ever conducted of women's lubricant use. It was a double-blind prospective study, which is science-speak for saying that neither the women themselves nor the scientists (my colleagues and I) knew which women received which lubricant. Sure, we had chosen the six lubricants that were being studied, but we didn't know which women got which one until after the study was over and every last woman had completed the study. We did this to enhance the study's validity and scientific objectivity, ensuring that no one involved would be biased toward a specific lubricant.

In our study, we found that when women used water-based or silicone-based lubricant during masturbation, vaginal sex, or anal sex, they rated these sex acts as more pleasurable and more satisfying compared to when they didn't use any lubricant. Does this mean that everyone should use lubricant every time they have sex? No, of course not. It does mean, however, that lubricant may have a positive role to play in many people's masturbation and partnered sex lives. Using lubricant during masturbation reduces friction between one's hand and genitals, or between one's vibrator and genitals. Using lubricant during penile-vaginal sex reduces friction between the penis and the vagina. And using lubricant during penile-anal sex reduces friction between those two parts. Too much friction can lead to uncomfortable or painful sex. If you've ever felt sore from sex, or found it almost uncomfortable to walk after particularly vigorous sex, you know what I'm talking about. Then again, too little friction during sex isn't ideal either; most people generally like at least a little bit of friction so they experience sensation during sex. When there's too little friction (perhaps because a woman is highly lubricated or she and her partner have used too much lubricant), both partners may say they don't feel much during sex. By experimenting with the amount of lubricant you use during masturbation or sex with a partner, you can find the right amount of friction for you. Think of it as a sexual balancing act.

In addition, I think of condoms as a type of sexual enhancement product. After all, if I told you that there was a product that could help relieve you of worries or stress about accidentally getting pregnant or getting an infection you don't want, I bet you would think that was pretty great. If you're feeling kind of "meh" or so-so about that, let's go back in time: imagine now that we're talking to people who lived a hundred years ago, a time when many women died in childbirth or had so many children that they spent their lives pregnant even when they didn't want to be. It was also a time, back before the invention of penicillin, when people often died of syphilis. Now imagine telling those women and men that they could plan their families, rather than risking pregnancy every time they had sex. Or that they could have sex with a very low risk of infection from syphilis. Now do you think condoms are a sexual enhancement product?

Sometimes I think we're so removed from how great modern medical technology is, and how far we've come, that we take products like condoms for granted. Even though condoms or other sheathlike barriers have been around for many generations, the modern condom is relatively new—as is our easy access to it, being able to purchase it in stores. The fact that, by using a condom, two people can share a sexual experience while putting their pregnancy and infection worries (mostly) to bed is nothing short of a miracle. Keep in mind, too, that as advanced as we are, condoms remain the one and only device that sexually active people can use to greatly reduce the risk of acquiring HIV. I have heard from many men and women who refuse to have sex without a condom, as well as from those who greatly prefer sex with a condom to sex without a condom, because they say they feel so much more relieved, relaxed, and confident about sex when they use one. That's why, at least in my view, condoms are key sexual enhancement products. This is not to mention that many of them now come with additional special features such as being textured (for example, ribbed or studded), flavored, or with a warming or cooling lubricant—though these special features are, as far as I'm concerned, the icing on an already delicious cake.

Need-to-Know Condom Info

Even if you haven't used condoms in years and it feels like a lifetime ago, it's worth reading through these basic tips about correct use of male condoms. You never know when you might use a condom again—or when a friend, son, or daughter might benefit from some helpful information from you.

Many people realize that they should check the condom's expiration date before they use it, carefully remove it from the package, and pinch the tip of the condom so as to leave a space at the top of it as it is unrolled all the way to the bottom of the penis. If you have that part down, you should do all right. Adding water-based or silicone-based lubricant to the outside of the condom after it's already on can make sex feel more natural for both partners. After ejaculation, the man should hold the condom against the base of his penis as he pulls out so as to make sure that the condom stays on and none of his semen and sperm drip out. These are the basics and many people get these right.

Unfortunately, while they may know how to put it on and remove it, many people use condoms incorrectly anyway. Too often, people start having sex and put a condom on midway through, or else they do the opposite: they start having sex with a condom on and then partway through, they remove the condom and continue with

> sex. Although there are some understandable reasons why people do this, it's not taking full advantage of the condom and it means putting yourself and your partner at potential risk for pregnancy and infection. To get the most bang for your condom buck, keep it on from the beginning to end of sex.

SEX TOY TOXIN NO-NOS

As sex toys have become more commonplace, more attention has turned to what they're made of. Many sex toys are made in China, and often, little information about their materials and manufacturing is available. Most sex toys come with little to no information about what they're made with, which is seriously frustrating for many women and men who want to make sure that what they're putting into or on their bodies is safe for them. As more sex toys are starting to become manufactured in the US and Canada where there are stricter guidelines for product manufacturing and package information, the public is beginning to have more information about sex toy materials.

As a general rule, I like to encourage people to steer clear of toys made with Jelly, which are often soft, flexible, and among the lowest-priced sex toys. These toys often contain what some believe are toxic materials. If left in warm cars or rooms too long, they can actually "melt" a little and change shape and emit a strong odor.

Sex toy materials that are generally considered safer to use and easier to clean (because they are less porous, whereas Jelly toys are more porous) are made of glass, hard plastic, or medical-grade silicone. That said, if you have allergies, make sure to select toys that are made of materials you're not allergic to. Although silicone allergies, for example, are uncommon, if you are allergic to silicone you will want to avoid using sex toys made with it.

If you're not sure what your sex toy is made of, ask. And if you're still not sure, or if you want to be on the safe side, slip a new lubricated condom over your sex toy when you use it. This will help serve as a barrier between whatever the toy is made of and your body.

SEX TOY HYGIENE

Most sex toys can be cleaned with soap and water while taking care to avoid getting the battery compartment wet. If your toy plugs into the wall, make sure it is unplugged before you attempt to wash it lest you risk electric shock (eek!). Some sex toy shops sell sex toy cleaner that can be used to spray the toy. This is one option but it isn't necessarily any better than using plain old soap and water. I'm not aware of any studies that have compared methods of sex toy cleaning so it's difficult to say how well different types of cleaning work or if one method is necessarily better than others.

If you're cleaning a nonvibrating dildo made of glass, hard plastic, or medical-grade silicone (and that doesn't have any batteries or motors inside it), you may be able to throw it in the dishwasher. Although this idea is difficult for many people to swallow, others find it an easy way to clean their sex toys.

After you've washed or otherwise cleaned your sex toy, leave it out to air dry. Bacteria love warm, wet environments, so getting your toy to a nice, dry state is a good goal. In our study, we found that most women cleaned their vibrator before or after use (and about 60 percent had cleaned both before and after use, at least sometimes).[6] However, almost 14 percent said that they had never cleaned their vibrator, either before or after use. Take a lesson from the 86 percent who do and give it a try, at least every now and then.

"HOW DO I USE THIS THING, ANYWAY?"

Many of my students and column readers have taken it upon themselves to go out and buy a vibrator or other sex toy, or they've received one as a gift from a partner, and then are left wondering how to use it. There are many ways to use sex toys and they vary greatly depending on the toy itself. For detailed information about how to use a variety of vibrators, dildos, cock rings, butt plugs, and more, check out my first book, *Because It Feels Good: A Complete Guide to Sexual Pleasure and Satisfaction,* where I devoted an entire chapter to the topic. Here, we'll focus on vibrators.

In our national vibrator study, we found that most women—84 percent—used their vibrators to stimulate the clitoris, whereas almost
two-thirds of women (64 percent) had used a vibrator inside the vagina.[7]
In addition, anecdotally I have heard from many women who use vibrators
to stimulate various parts of their body including their breasts, labia, mons,
and the area around the anal opening. Some women own a separate vibrator or dildo for anal penetration (it's a good idea to keep this as a separate
toy so as not to transfer bacteria or viruses between the vagina and anus).
The short answer, then, to "How do I use a vibrator?" is "However you
want" or "However turns you on"—as long as it's in a safe way, of course.
Some women perform oral sex on a vibrator or dildo, though I don't recommend turning the vibrator on if you're doing this on the off chance that
it will hurt your teeth or jostle any dental fillings you might have.

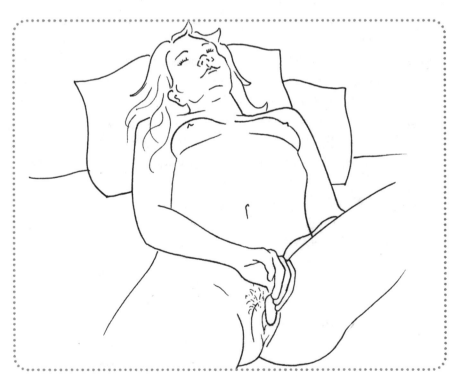

**Some women hold a small vibrator, such as a Silver Bullet vibrator, to their clitoris for
pleasurable sexual stimulation.**

Some vibrators are particularly well suited for clitoral use. Silver Bullet vibrators are small and made to be held against the clitoris; they are not to be inserted into the vagina. For safety reasons, you should avoid placing any parts of sex toys that look like motors, cords, or battery compartments into the vagina. Toys that have sharp edges are best avoided, or, if you have one, at least place a condom over it before inserting it into the vagina or holding it against the clitoris. While stimulating their clitoris with a vibrator, some women simply hold it up to their clitoris. Others press the toy against the clitoris in a pulsating or rhythmic pattern. Some women feel that their clitoris is too sensitive for direct stimulation and prefer instead to place the vibrator somewhat near, but not directly on, the clitoris.

For vaginal stimulation, some women insert a vaginal vibrator and lie there, perhaps squeezing the muscles around the vagina to tighten around the vibrator. Some women use an "in and out" motion with the vibrator. Others treat the vibrator as if it were a penis and might "mount" it in different ways, such as getting into a woman-on-top position, or else they might lie facedown on the bed and press the vibrator into the bed with their vagina. Certain sex toys have suction cup bases that allow women to stick the vibrator or dildo to a wall or bathtub (in cases in which the vibrator is waterproof). This can make for a variety of fun sex positions, including standing up and bending over against the vibrator. G Spot vibrators (which are often curved on one end) can be used internally for vaginal G Spot stimulation or they can be held against the clitoris for clitoral stimulation.

If you're using a sex toy with a partner, tap into your creativity. Remember: vibrators can be used in many different ways. Some sex toy shops sell small vibrators along with massage gloves. Simply slip the vibrator into the massage glove and your or your partner's hand becomes an intense vibrating machine! If your sex partner is a guy, you might want to massage the vibrator up and down the shaft of his penis. Some men find that vibration is too intense up around the head of the penis. The base of the penis, particularly around the scrotum, is a well-loved vibration spot for many men and perhaps one reason why vibrating penis rings (cock rings) are so popular among men and their partners. And while vibrators can be used around a man's anal opening or inside of it (as long as it has a wide, flared base to keep the sex toy from being sucked upward and out of reach), it's best not to put a toy in one's butt if it's been in the vagina or on the vulva, and vice versa. Keep anal and vaginal/vulva toys separate and buy your own "butt toys" for anal pleasuring.

Finally, before you start to use the vibrator, consider using a lubricant with it. In our national study, only 41 percent of vibrator users said that they had ever used lubricant along with their vibrator[8]—a shame, considering how lubricant use can enhance pleasure and satisfaction while also helping increase comfort and perhaps reduce the risk of tearing. Silicone-based lubricants cannot be used with all sex toys, as they can make silicone-based sex toys slightly more porous, making them more difficult to keep clean. Water-based lubricants, however, can be used with a wide range of sex toys and are a great option for sex toy play alone or with a partner.

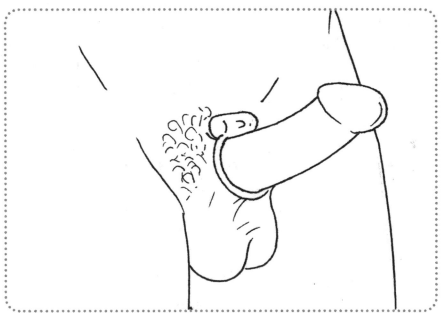

Vibrating c-rings can be worn around a man's penis. Positioning the vibrating portion on the top of the base (closest to his lower abdomen) can make clitoral stimulation easier during face-to-face sex positions such as missionary and woman on top.

DIY Sex Toys: What's Safe Versus What Will Make You Sorry

Human beings are wonderful, creative creatures. We've discovered fire, invented the wheel, and even created magical little devices to carry thousands of digital songs with us, ready to be listened to wherever and whenever we want. It's pretty impressive when you think about it, isn't it? However, sometimes human creativity and inventiveness get people in trouble. With all the great sex toys on the market, there's no need to put anything unsafe inside your body for sexual purposes. People have wound up in the emergency room with everything from light bulbs to beer bottles stuck inside their rectum. Worryingly, several young girls have been admitted to hospital emergency rooms with abdominal complaints and/or fever, only to have it discovered that they had inserted batteries into their vagina and left them there. Batteries are dangerous to the vagina and can cause very serious health problems requiring hospitalization. Make sure to keep batteries out of your child's reach and to give your children age-appropriate information about how to take care of their bodies. This is also an important take-home message that's relevant to shopping for and using vibrators. Avoid buying a sex toy that has a battery compartment positioned in a place that would involve inserting it into the vagina. If the compartment were to come open while the toy was inside your vagina, the battery could potentially dislodge and be inside the vagina. Similarly, try to use your sex toys safely—again, making sure to keep all batteries and battery compartments outside the vaginal canal.

"SO, WHAT DO YOU THINK ABOUT . . ."

Although many women and men use sex toys, people sometimes feel shy or uncertain about how to talk with their sexual partner about their desire to add sex toys to their partnered sex. Some women worry that their partner will feel threatened or intimidated by the idea of using a vibrator. Some men worry that their partners will think they're perverted. According to a recent study that our Indiana University research team conducted and published in a 2011 issue of the *Journal of Sex and Marital Therapy*, the vast majority of American men and women feel positively about women's vibrator use. For example, 74 percent of women and 82 percent of men felt that vibrator use could enhance a woman's relationship and about two-thirds of women and men felt that vibrator use could take the pressure off a woman's partner to give her an orgasm. If you've been wondering how your partner would feel about you using a vibrator together (or alone), chances are your partner would jump right on board.

Many women who partner with men worry in particular that their boyfriends or husbands will feel threatened or intimidated by her vibrator use, but that's rarely the case. In our study, 63 percent of women and 70 percent of men ages eighteen to sixty in the US thought that a woman's vibrator use was not intimidating to her partner.[9] One of the important take-home messages I get from these data is that men feel even more positively about vibrator use than many women realize. By talking about these issues with your partner, you will get a chance to learn more about how they feel about using sex toys together—and you may feel closer to your partner just by opening up, sharing your feelings, and finding out what turns your partner on. Sometimes, people feel too shy to share their sexual interests with a partner. With a long-term relationship partner, they may not want to "rock the boat" and risk changing an otherwise good (but not great) sex life. In newer relationships or friends-with-benefits situations, people may not know how to approach their partner, or else they may feel embarrassed to share that level of intimacy. However, the benefits of having a more satisfying sex life can be well worth the risk. I say, go for it!

To start a conversation about vibrators with your partner, try saying something like

- "What do you think about vibrators?"
- "You know, I like using my vibrator when I'm alone, but I've often thought it would be fun to use with you. What do you think about that?"
- "Have you ever wondered what it would be like for us to try using sex toys together?"

• "In this book I'm reading, it talked about how more than half of American women have used a vibrator—and that most of them have used one with a partner. It got me thinking that I'd like to use one with you. What do you think?"

Who knows? By starting a simple conversation about sex toys, you might just begin a new and exciting chapter of your sex life.

Greening Your Sex Play

In this age of greener transportation and farm-to-table food, I would be remiss if I didn't at least mention the many ways in which people try to green their sex play. Although the "greenest" way to have sex is au naturel, let's face it: few of us do it that way. Most of us like having sex in air-conditioned or heated homes and most of us use, or have used, any number of products that we think make for better sex (condoms, lubricants, sex toys, music playing in the background, candles lit, etc.). That doesn't mean we can't do our best to be greener where we can. Here are some options for greening your sex play:

Sex Toys

There are an increasing number of ecofriendly sex toys available on the market, including sex toys made from recycled materials, vibrators that use rechargeable batteries, solar-powered vibrators, dildos made of hardwood, glass dildos and vibrators, and a windup vibrator called the Earth Angel. After you wind it up for a minute or two, it offers a surprisingly intense vibration. Having a wider range of available nontoxic sex toy materials (like glass, hardwood, or plastic) is important, as it gives consumers more choices than sex toys made with Jelly, which often contain PVCs. Some women go the DIY route by using lubricated condom-covered zucchini or cucumbers as vaginal dildos (produce should never go into the vagina without a condom over it; also produce should never be inserted into the anus, as it can easily get sucked up inside the anus, out of reach). Long, thin, smooth candles can also double as vaginal dildos (again, it's better to cover them with a lubricated condom) or vaginal dilators.

Sex Toy Recycling

Some sex toy shops and web sites also offer sex toy recycling promotions. Popular sex boutique Early to Bed in Chicago, Illinois (www.early2bed.com), and Love Honey in the UK are two shops that are well known for their sex toy recycling efforts. Ask your local shop if they recycle sex toys. Learn more about LoveHoney's program, which they call the Rabbit Amnesty program, online at http://www.lovehoney.co.uk/rabbit-amnesty.

Lubricants

Look for lubricants made with organic ingredients, such as Good Clean Love. Of course, you can also green your lubrication by spending more time in foreplay to build up the body's own natural vaginal lubrication or by using saliva as lubricant. That said, some research suggests that saliva may get in the way of sperm movement, making it less than ideal for couples trying to conceive. Another downside to using saliva as a lubricant is that some research shows that women who are prone to recurrent yeast infections may be at greater risk when saliva gets on their genitals, such as by receiving oral sex or when saliva is used as a lubricant during penile-vaginal sex. Finally, another way to be greener about your lubricant use is to keep a small bowl of room-temperature water by your bedside. Once you apply water-based lubricant during sex, if you feel it starting to dry out (as water-based lubricant often does because it absorbs into the vaginal and vulva tissue), dab some water on your genitals to revive the lubricant rather than reapplying even more lubricant (this is the "reduce" part of the "reduce, reuse, recycle" strategy).

Lingerie

Why buy new when you can shop vintage? Check out local shops to see what beautiful old vintage lingerie you can find, such as sexy slips, negligees, corsets, and robes.

—Making It Easy—

65. What to do if . . . your genitals go numb from vibrator play

Genital numbness from vibrator play is rare. In our national vibrator study, the vast majority of women who used vibrators—83.5 percent of them—said they had never experienced any genital numbness in connection with vibrator use.[10] Of the 16.5 percent who had, most of them said it had happened only once or a few times. A small number said it had happened every time. When genital numbness did occur, it usually lasted only briefly (for less than five minutes or for less than an hour).

If you experience genital numbness in connection with vibrator use, there are a few things you can try. You can stop using the vibrator—at least until you have a chance to ask your health care provider about it. You can also shop around for a lower-intensity vibrator or one with a multispeed dial so that you can change the intensity based on your individual preferences or desires. Some women enjoy the power of a high-intensity vibrator but find that it's too much for direct contact with their genitals. Rather than holding the vibrator directly to their vulva, they place a soft towel, blanket, or piece of clothing in between the vibrator and their vulva or clitoris. Other women like having the vibrator directly pressed against the clitoris or another vulva part and find that applying a generous amount of water-based lubricant is enough to reduce the friction and make vibrator use more comfortable. If you have ongoing issues or genital numbness or other side effects that concern you, or if the numbness or other side effects are severe or bother you or you simply have questions, please check in with a health care provider.

66. What to do if . . . a sex toy gets "lost" in your or his body

If a sex toy has gone missing in action inside your vagina, try not to panic. The vagina is a small, discrete space and the cervix at the other end of it is too small for a sex toy to pass through. It's even too small for tampons to pass through, which is why it's such a safe space to put things like tampons and the birth control ring (NuvaRing)—it's not going anywhere.

> ### You'll Never Look at a Cucumber Sandwich the Same Way Again
>
> Several years ago, Durex (a major global condom brand) got into the vibrator business—and when they did, they created a great video on the topic that went viral. Don't worry: I won't give anything away here except to say that it involves a cucumber sandwich. Search "Durex sandwich video" or "Durex cucumber sandwich video" to find it on YouTube.

So if a sex toy such as a vaginal ball or a small dildo has slipped out of reach inside your vagina, try to relax. Take deep breaths and, as you're able to, slip a lubricated finger slowly inside your vagina, feeling around for the object that has gone MIA. Chances are that you will be able to find it and slowly remove it. If a partner is with you, he or she can do the same thing by slowly inserting a finger and carefully removing the toy. This can also be done if you're using a condom during vaginal intercourse and it slips off. If for some reason you cannot find the sex toy or condom, please check in with your health care provider and let him or her know that there's an object in there and you need their help getting it out. Believe it or not, this happens fairly often: gynecologists often help with removing forgotten tampons, condoms that have slipped off, and—yes—at least in one case, a vibrator that a woman had left in her vagina for more than a year (this last case was a very difficult situation that was dangerous to her health, which is why it is important to seek help immediately rather than leave an object where it doesn't belong).

If a sex toy has gone missing inside the anus and rectum, it's another story. It is far easier for objects to slip far enough inside that they are difficult to remove on one's own. If the object is sharp, breakable, or has pointed edges (like a light bulb, bottle, broom handle, or sharp sex toy—and yes, every single one of these are objects that doctors have removed from patients' rectums in the emergency room), don't even try to remove it yourself. Call for an ambulance or ask your partner to drive you to the emergency room. You don't want to risk hurting yourself or your partner in an effort to remove it. If the toy or object is smooth and not breakable, you may be able to try to remove it on your own. However, don't try too hard or too long; if you are unable to remove it within a few minutes, even after relaxation, the best course of action is to get yourself or your partner to the emergency room. Going forward, only insert sex toys or other objects into the anus and rectum if they have a wide, flared base or a ring that one can slip one's finger through to hold on to it. Both of these toy features make it far more difficult for the sex toy to slip upward and out of reach.

67. What to do if . . . you find out that your roommate or partner "borrowed" your vibrator while you were away

If your partner borrowed your sex toy and it's one that you are using together anyway, and you have already been tested for STIs and are comfortable with each other's STI status, then it may not be that big a deal. Keep in mind, though, that if you or your partner has an STI, it is possible to pass it to one another through sex toy use. Clean it anyway.

If your roommate "borrowed" your sex toy, this is likely a more serious concern. Unless you have sex with your roommate (which of course some people do), you won't be used to sharing sexual fluids with one another. You probably have no idea what your roommate's STI status is or whether he or she has other infections or germs that you don't want in or around your genitals. Some sex toys are more porous than others, which means that some harbor bacteria and viruses more easily than others—even after cleaning. If you absolutely cannot afford to replace your sex toy and your roommate won't pony up the cash to replace it, you could potentially wash it with soap and hot water and then place a new condom over it before you use it again. While washing, try not to get water near the battery pack, and if it's the kind of vibrator that plugs into the wall, make sure it's unplugged while you're washing it. However, my best advice is to throw the sex toy out, or recycle it if there's a sex toy recycling program available to you, and get a brand new one. Also, keep it in a locked box if you don't trust your roommate. And at the next opportunity, get a new roommate who is more respectful of your belongings and more attentive to health issues.

68. What to do if . . . his penis is bruised
after using a cock ring

Generally speaking, many health care providers recommend wearing cock rings no more than twenty minutes at a time and taking them off if a man begins to experience discomfort, pain, or bruising. Most of the time, cock ring play goes off without a hitch. Every once in a blue moon, however, a man will have pain or bruising from wearing a cock ring and it is serious enough to appear to cause erection problems or other health issues. After all, cock rings constrict blood flow to the genitals. Done in a mild way, that's not such a risky thing. But if blood flow is seriously restricted to the penis, or if it's done for a long time, that's dangerous. Any time a man experiences pain or bruising on his penis or scrotum, he should check in with a health care provider (such as a urologist) as soon as he can—even on an emergency room basis (particularly for genital pain or dark or extensive bruising). It's always better to be safe than sorry. A man only gets one penis in life and it's up to him—and his sexual partners—to care for it.

69. What to do if . . . he asks you to use
a prostate toy on him

Some women are open minded and enthusiastic about using a prostate toy on a male partner. And some women feel strongly against it, or even squeamish about it. Many women are probably somewhere in the middle: open to it, curious about it, but full of questions.

As a rule, I like to encourage couples to consider each other's requests before saying no (and often before saying yes). It's okay to think about something before doing it. If he asks you to try a prostate toy on him and the idea is new to you, it's okay to say something like, "I've never done that before, but I'm open to the idea if it's something you'd like. Let's talk about it some more." This gives you a chance to ask questions, such as what kind of toy he's interested in trying (for example, a butt plug, anal beads, a prostate-specific sex toy, dildo, or strap-on) and how he'd like it used (gently, roughly, as part of role play?). Talking about it before trying it also gives you both a chance to determine whether there's anything else you need to make your sexual exploration easier or more pleasurable. For example, any time you're inserting something into the anus or rectum, it's wise to use water-based or silicone-based lubricant. In our lubricant study, we found that the women rated water-based lubricant slightly higher than silicone-based lubricant for anal sex. However, both received very high ratings in terms of making sex feel pleasurable and satisfying, so to some degree it's a matter of personal preference.

If you decide to march forward into the land of prostate play, keep a few things in mind:

• **Prostate play** has nothing to do with sexual orientation. Plenty of straight men like prostate play, as do plenty of gay and bisexual men. Then again, some men in each sexual orientation group don't like prostate play. It's highly individual.

• **Start small.** If one or both of you is new to prostate stimulation, it may be easiest and most comfortable to start with something small such as a finger covered with a well-lubricated condom or a thin dildo that has a very wide base (so that it doesn't get sucked up inside the anus and rectum out of reach).

• **Go slowly at first.** Even with water-based lubricant, it can take time, patience, and a great deal of relaxation to insert something into a man's anus and rectum.

For more detailed information about anal play, including prostate play, check out my e-book *The Good in Bed Guide to Anal Pleasuring* (www.goodinbed.com).

70. What to do if . . . you get cuts or tears during sex

It's not unusual for women to occasionally notice very light pink blood stains on toilet paper when they pee sometime after sex or on their underwear within twenty-four hours after sex. This can be a sign of having experienced "microtears"—very small cuts or tears, possibly not even noticeable to the naked eye—inside the vagina or on the vulva itself. One way to reduce the risk of getting cuts or tears during sex is to spend significant time in foreplay, giving the body enough time to warm up and produce sufficient amounts of vaginal lubrication. Remember: vaginal lubrication can help reduce friction and protect the vagina.

A second strategy is to start out slow during sex, as it gives you a chance to find your groove before adopting a faster pace. Some women also find that by choosing positions, such as woman on top, that allow them to assume greater control over how fast or slow or deep or shallow the penetration is, they can reduce the likelihood of vaginal cuts or tears. Finally, consider using a store-bought lubricant to decrease friction even more, making sex more comfortable and pleasurable. In our 2011 lubricant study, 22 percent of women said that they used lubricants during vaginal intercourse in order to reduce the risk of tearing. For anal sex, this figure was more than double, at 53 percent of women. If you continue to experience vaginal cuts or tears during masturbation or sex with a partner, even after trying these or other strategies, let your health care provider know. Some medical conditions or low-estrogen states (such as breastfeeding or menopause) can cause the vaginal tissue or vulvar skin to be thinner and more fragile, making women more vulnerable to tearing.

70. What to do if . . . a condom breaks or slips off during sex

If this happens before a man has ejaculated, it's probably not a big deal. Is it ideal? Of course not. However, if he hasn't yet ejaculated, the chances of pregnancy risk are extremely low. The chances of infection risk are increased the more your genitals touch each other, but you also can't go back and rewrite history to keep the condom on. The best you can do is make sure to get tested for STIs and try to do a better job keeping the condom on the next time. If the condom break or slip isn't noticed until after your partner has ejaculated, it's a bigger deal with more significant risks. If the condom was your one and only form of birth control, then you may be at risk of pregnancy. You might want to consider getting emergency contraception (EC, also known as the "morning-after pill") to reduce your risk of pregnancy. EC is most effective when taken within three days of unprotected sex. Again, follow up with STI testing. You will want to ask your health care provider how soon you can be tested for STIs such as chlamydia or gonorrhea, as it depends on the types of lab tests that a particular clinic uses. Some health care providers recommend coming in for testing several days after unprotected sex, whereas others advise waiting about two weeks for general STI testing and a month for an HIV test; although not everyone who has HIV will test positive one month after exposure, most HIV-positive individuals will.

The Condom You Might Never Have Heard Of

Many people in the US have never heard of the female condom—and if they have heard of it, they may never have seen one. They are rarely carried in drugstores or pharmacies. Those who do use them often order them online. However, female condoms are more widely available in countries outside the US, particularly as part of programs that work to empower women to take charge of their sexual and reproductive health and insist on condom use. In some ways, female condoms resemble pouches or baggies. The closed end is inserted into the vagina, which means that using them requires some degree of comfort touching one's genitals. The open end frames a woman's vaginal entrance so that her male partner can insert his penis into her vagina and only come into contact with the female condom (not her vagina itself). In this way, it serves as a barrier between his penis and her genitals. Even though the name of the female condom makes it sound as though it's used only by women, in fact some men who have sex with men use it during anal sex. Used in this way, the pouch end is inserted partly into the anus and rectum. To learn more about the female condom, check out www.avert.org or www.plannedparenthood.org.

71. What to do if . . . you run out of condoms but desperately want sex one more time and aren't on birth control

Many doctors, nurses, and health educators would tell you to control your desires, put your pants back on, and forget it: there is no safe way to have sex "just one time" if you're not on birth control. They're right: if you're looking to greatly reduce your risk of pregnancy and infections, condoms are the way to go. That said, I live in the real world and I know that millions of people have sex that puts them at risk, even when they know better. People take chances. If you find yourself in this situation, the best case scenario truly is to take a deep breath and try to resist. Do something else sexual that helps you to feel good and satisfies your desires but doesn't put you at risk. Straight couples (men and women together) are often focused on vaginal sex as if it were the only way to feel good sexually. Same-sex couples (gay men and lesbians) are often far more creative in bed because their sex lives don't revolve around penis-in-vagina sex. If you're in a heterosexual relationship, take a lesson and expand your idea of sex. It can be just as gratifying to masturbate each other or to masturbate in front of one another while kissing. Oral sex is another option; there is no pregnancy risk involved with oral sex, although there is still some risk of passing STI (however, it's a lower-risk activity than unprotected vaginal sex).

If you decide to throw caution to the wind and have vaginal or anal sex, even without a condom, at least ask him to pull out before he ejaculates. If you're not sure he's able to, then you might proceed with a few moments of intercourse and then, if you're on top, get off him (or have him pull out) and bring him to orgasm some other way, such as with your hands. If you can keep his semen out of your vagina, you will reduce your risk of infection and pregnancy. It's not the ideal situation but as far as the real world goes, it's better than nothing. And of course, make sure to follow up with appropriate STI and HIV testing.

Get Local

Find an HIV testing site near you by visiting www.hivtest.org. Local-area STI testing can be found through www.findstdtest.org, websites that are services of the US Centers for Disease Control and Prevention. You can learn more about HIV and STI by calling the CDC at 1-800-CDC-INFO.

Sex Smarts Quiz

1. Which toy should silicone lubricant not be used with?
   a. A Silver Bullet vibrator made of hard plastic
   b. A glass dildo
   c. A vibrator made of medical-grade silicone
   d. None of the above
2. Which of the following is the best advice when it comes to anal and vaginal toys?
   a. Vibrators are best inserted in the vagina first and the anus second
   b. It is safest to insert a vibrator in the anus first and the vagina second
   c. Vaginal and anal toys shouldn't be mixed. Buy a separate one for each activity.
   d. All of the above
3. Most women use vibrators to stimulate their
   a. Clitoris
   b. Mons
   c. Vagina
   d. Labia

Answers
   1. c
   2. c
   3. a

Chapter 8
Sexploration: Giving Fantasies a Whirl

What do Americans do in their private sex lives? How often do people have sex? And when they have sex, what exactly are they doing? These questions form the backdrop for many of the emails and letters I receive from readers of my sex advice columns. Given how much secrecy surrounds sex, it's no wonder that so many people would like to move sex conversations out of the dark and into the light.

Scientists have similar questions about sex too, though often for different reasons. We want to know what kinds of sexual behaviors people engage in, how often, and how they protect themselves from STI and pregnancy (if they do). After all, understanding human sexual behavior matters to our nation's health. If we can better understand what people do sexually, doctors, nurses, health educators, teachers, and parents can provide better—and more relevant—sexual health information to the people who need it.

Safer Sexploration

If you're having sex with someone you don't know well—whether it's someone you meet out at a bar or party or someone you connect with at a sex club—please consider making it as safe as possible. Use a condom. If you think using a condom with someone you don't know well is the obvious choice that anyone would make, think again. In our national sex survey, our research team found that teenagers were the best condom users of anyone. A total of 84 percent of young men and 89 percent of young women said that they used a condom the last time they had vaginal sex with a casual partner. That's great news, considering what a high STI risk group teenagers are in (not to mention unintended pregnancy).

Surprisingly, condom use wasn't nearly as common among

older adults who were having casual sex. Only 53 percent of men and 42 percent of women ages twenty-five to twenty-nine used a condom during vaginal sex with their most recent casual sex partner.[1] For those in their thirties, 58 percent of men and 31 percent of women whose most recent vaginal sex was with a casual partner said they used a condom. Adults in their forties were even less likely to use a condom with a casual partner: only 36 percent of men and 20 percent of women said they used one. Sex shouldn't be like Russian roulette. Keep condoms in your wallet and/or purse and insist on using them—especially if you don't know your partner's STI history, if you're not ready to become pregnant, or if you suspect your partner may have, or may have recently had, sex partners other than you.

How Sex Has Changed

In our National Survey of Sexual Health and Behavior, we discovered that one of the biggest recent changes to occur in Americans' sexual lives has to do with anal sex. In an earlier survey of sex in America that was conducted in the 1990s, it was found that as many as 20 to 25 percent of Americans in some age groups had had anal sex.[2-4] In our study, which was conducted close to twenty years later, we found that far more people had engaged in anal sex, which was reported by

- 10 percent of men and 20 percent of women ages eighteen to nineteen
- 24 percent of men and 40 percent of women ages twenty to twenty-four
- 45 percent of men and 46 percent of women ages twenty-five to twenty-nine
- 45 percent of men and 40 percent of women in their thirties
- 43 percent of men and 41 percent of women in their forties
- 40 percent of men and 35 percent of women in their fifties

192 Sex Made Easy

- 27 percent of men and 30 percent of women in their sixties
- 14 percent of men and 21 percent of women ages seventy or older

Of course, many of these people may have only tried anal sex once or twice and others may have engaged in it more often. Regardless, this is a massive shift in sexual behavior and it's important. If we all kept believing, based on outdated scientific data, that only 20 percent or so of Americans had ever tried anal sex, we would be missing out on important opportunities to educate people about an increasingly common sexual behavior. This matters for reasons of health and pleasure.

If we fail to understand how common anal sex is, we're missing the boat on understanding more about HPV-related anal cancer (HPV can be transmitted during anal sex and has been linked to a number of cancers, including anal cancer). Other STIs including chlamydia and gonorrhea can also be transmitted during anal sex, and if doctors and their patients don't talk more openly about sex, including anal sex, that's a problem. If you have ever had anal sex, let your health care provider know so he or she can decide whether or not to offer you rectal STI testing (chlamydia and gonorrhea in the anus/rectum cannot be detected from vaginal testing, so separate testing is often recommended).

MORE PLEASURABLE PLAY

As I've said before, there are health reasons for studying changes in sexual behavior and there are also reasons related to sexual pleasure and satisfaction. People who decide to engage in anal sex can benefit from learning about ways to be safer but also to have a more enjoyable experience. Knowing that nearly half of women and men in some age groups have had anal sex reminds me, as a sex educator, to talk and write more often about anal sex so that if people want to try it, they have enough information to enhance their experience. If part of your sexploration involves anal play, I would encourage you to read a book focused on anal pleasuring, such as *The Good in Bed Guide to Anal Pleasuring* (which I wrote and is available at www.goodinbed.com), for detailed tips and techniques. Among the most important pieces of advice you should know for safer, more pleasurable anal play are

• **Start small and slow.** A finger covered with a lubricated condom (along with a little extra water-based lubricant)—or a small condom-covered and lubricated butt plug—is a fine size to start with.

• **There are two sets of muscles inside the anus.** One is under voluntary control, meaning that you can relax it at will. Another is not under voluntary control, which means that you can't "make" yourself relax it. If your body isn't relaxing on its own and penetration feels difficult or impossible, try to breathe deeply and give it a few moments. If it still doesn't work, try again another day (or not).

• **Lubrication is key.** Unlike the vagina, the anus doesn't make its own lubricant. If anal penetration is in the cards, adding your own water-based lubricant can make a world of difference in terms of comfort and pleasure.

• **There are many ways to play.** When people think about anal sex, they often think about a penis going into a person's anus and rectum. Yet anal play involves a number of different activities, including stroking or licking the area around the anal opening (without penetration), playing with anal sex toys, holding a vibrator against the anal opening (again, without penetration), and more.

• **If you're going to switch, keep it clean.** If you're planning to go between vaginal and anal penetration (or vice versa), clean whatever it is you're using and/or use a new condom. Don't use the same sex toy for both places, and if a male partner's penis is involved, use a clean condom for vaginal sex and a clean condom for anal sex (change condoms in between).

• **Steer clear of anal desensitizers.** If you see products for anal numbing or desensitizing, my advice is do not use them. Numbing your body to pain isn't often advised. After all, pain and discomfort are your body's way of saying "stop." In my opinion, if you're going to have anal penetration, it's a better idea to know when your body wants you to stop.

• **Respect each other's boundaries.** Not everyone is into anal sex and not everyone who tries it wants to do it again. For some women and men, the anus and rectum are "exit only" (as many of my female college students like to say). That's OK. Even if you try anal sex and like it, it's your right to do it when you want to and to say no to anal sex when you're not feeling like it.

Of course, anal sex isn't the only thing about sex that has changed in the past couple of decades. As mentioned in an earlier chapter, sex toy use has changed too, with more than half of women and almost half of men now having used vibrators.

As society changes, sex changes. By staying up to date with what's common, what's not, and what people do, we get a glimpse of sex that can help us ask questions about our own sex lives. I certainly don't believe that people should feel pressured to change their sex lives to be more like their neighbors (or their best friends or exes or anyone else). However, sometimes knowing what other people do gives people something to think about or provokes healthy conversation between sexual partners.

VARIETY IS THE SPICE OF SEX

Discovering how sex has changed is one important aspect of sex research. Another is looking at how sex stays the same and looking at it from new angles.

Case in point: if there's one thing that hasn't changed much throughout human history, it's that sex remains diverse and varied. Even though people don't talk openly about the many ways they express themselves sexually, we know that men and women entertain themselves with a number of sex acts behind closed doors. For example, people engage in closed-mouth kissing, open-mouth (tongue) kissing, cunnilingus (oral sex performed on a woman), fellatio (oral sex performed on a man), masturbation, mutual masturbation, sex toy play, breast touching, breast licking, anal touching, anal licking (analingus), vaginal intercourse, anal intercourse, stripping, and much more.

The more things change, the more they stay (relatively) the same. Just as the *Kama Sutra* detailed a host of sex positions, our sex study documented forty-one different combinations of sexual behavior that the men and women in the study engaged in during their most recent sexual experience. We also found that sexual variety is linked to men's and women's orgasm. For example, 92 percent of men who reported having engaged in just one sex act during their most recent sexual experience reported having had an orgasm. However, 97 percent of those men who reported having engaged in five sex acts reported having an orgasm, as did 100 percent of the (small number of) men who engaged in six sex acts during their most recent sexual experience.[5]

We saw a similar—but more striking—pattern among women. Only 55 percent of women who reported having engaged in one sex act during their most recent sexual experience said that they had an orgasm. In contrast, orgasm was reported by 60 percent of women who had engaged in two sex acts, 78 percent of women who had engaged in three sex acts, 76 percent of women who engaged in four sex acts, 89 percent of those who engaged in five sex acts, and all of the (again, very few) women who had engaged in six sex acts during their most recent sexual experience.

Does this mean that if you engage in more sex acts you will be guaranteed to have an orgasm? No, probably not (I have yet to come across anything that guarantees orgasm for women or men). It may be that sexual experimentation and exploration help people find what "works" for them and help them orgasm. Or it may be that people who keep trying lots of different things sexually are unusually determined to have or give an orgasm—sort of an "I won't rest until it happens!" strategy (which can be sweet or annoying depending on your perspective).

My take on sex comes down to being aware of what you want and communicating about it with your partner. There is probably some truth to the idea that sexual exploration is linked to easier orgasms. After all, if you try different types of sexual stimulation, you are likely to hit upon something that feels good for one or both partners. It may also be that people who try more things sexually are also people who spend more time having sex. Rather than a quickie approach to sex, they may take their time to develop sex play that works well for both partners.

The Best Laundry List You'll Ever Meet

Some time ago, a reader of the *Kinsey Confidential* sex columns I write asked if I knew of any lists consisting of sexual behaviors. He and his wife wanted to have a more adventurous sex life, weren't sure where to start, and wondered if such a list existed. Their idea was that if they saw a list of sexual behaviors, they could go through the list and decide what they wanted to try together. I didn't know of such a list but I felt inspired by the idea and consequently wrote one and posted it to my blog with the following instructions:

Below you'll find a list of more than sixty things people can do sexually with a partner. You and your partner might enjoy using this list to find out what you'd like to try doing with each other. Simply print two copies of the list. Each of you can then privately complete your list and, after you're both done, compare your responses. As you go through the list, you may find it helpful to talk not only about the things that you both want to try, but also about the types of sex where you differ. Is one person a "little" interested whereas the other is "very" interested in that activity? If so, is the person who is a little interested willing to explore under certain circumstances that might make the sexual behavior more appealing? Enjoy your exploration!

Mark each of the following activities with a number to indicate how interested you are in trying it (0 = Not interested, 1 = A little interested, 2 = Somewhat interested, 3 = Very interested).

☐ 1. Masturbating in front of each other

☐ 2. Vaginal intercourse

☐ 3. Mutual oral sex ("69")

☐ 4. Anal intercourse

☐ 5. Oral-anal sex ("rimming")

☐ 6. Role-playing (doctor/nurse, prisoner/warden, teacher/student, etc.)

☐ 7. Using a sex toy on yourself

☐ 8. Using a sex toy on your partner

☐ 9. Vaginal fisting

☐ 10. Anal fisting

☐ 11. Stripping for your partner

☐ 12. Your partner stripping for you

☐ 13. Having sex on a beach

☐ 14. Having sex under the stars

☐ 15. Having sex in the car while parked on the side of a road

☐ 16. Having a threesome

☐ 17. Having sex in front of other people at a sex club

☐ 18. Watching other people have sex at a sex club

☐ 19. Hiring a prostitute/sex worker together
    (in a place where it's legal, of course)

☐ 20. Eating food off your partner's body

☐ 21. Having your partner eat food off your body

☐ 22. Whipping your partner (safely and consensually)

☐ 23. Being whipped by your partner (again, safely and consensually)

☐ 24. Tying or otherwise binding your partner

☐ 25. Being tied up or bound by your partner

☐ 26. Engaging in a golden shower (peeing on one another)

☐ 27. Giving or receiving a facial (ejaculating on a partner's face)

☐ 28. Breast touching or massage

☐ 29. Bathing together

☐ 30. Making a homemade sex tape

☐ 31. Sending each other sexy photos

☐ 32. Sending each other sexy texts

☐ 33. Having sex while in the shower

- [ ] 34. Having sex in a cheap motel room
- [ ] 35. Having sex in a luxurious hotel room or suite
- [ ] 36. Licking champagne off your partner's body
- [ ] 37. Asking your partner to lick champagne off your body
- [ ] 38. Hiring someone to photograph you having sex together
- [ ] 39. Calling in sick from work and staying home to make love
- [ ] 40. Having a simultaneous orgasm (orgasm at the same time)
- [ ] 41. Prostate stimulation
- [ ] 42. Grooming or shaving each other's pubic hair
- [ ] 43. Wearing sexy lingerie
- [ ] 44. Spending at least thirty minutes having foreplay
- [ ] 45. Making out for an hour without touching each other's genitals
- [ ] 46. Dry humping
- [ ] 47. Having sex three times in one day
- [ ] 48. Having sex every day for a month
- [ ] 49. Reading erotic stories to each other
- [ ] 50. Writing love poems for one another
- [ ] 51. Writing an erotic story together
- [ ] 52. Squeezing your and/or your partner's nipples
- [ ] 53. Spanking or being spanked
- [ ] 54. Acting like a gender other than the one you identify with
- [ ] 55. Kissing your partner's entire body from the top of their head to the bottom of their feet (or being kissed all over by your partner)
- [ ] 56. Licking your partner's body
- [ ] 57. Watching porn together
- [ ] 58. Nipple clamping
- [ ] 59. Axillary intercourse (penis is thrust through a partner's armpit opening)
- [ ] 60. Penile intercourse between the thighs (but not in the vagina or anus)
- [ ] 61. Penile intercourse between the breasts
- [ ] 62. Performing oral sex
- [ ] 63. Receiving oral sex
- [ ] 64. Masturbating each other
- [ ] 65. Receiving oral sex with your underwear still on

Humans Aren't the Only Ones Who Like Variety

Sometimes we humans like to think we invented sex. Yet most animal species engage in some form of mating in order to reproduce. Many are just as inventive as we humans are. Numerous animals engage in same-sex sexual behavior and some have long-standing pair bonds (the animal version of close relationships) with animals of their same sex. Some animals also seem to exchange sex for objects (such as pebbles for one's nest): what some describe as animals' version of prostitution. Others have been observed using objects (such as sticks) for genital stimulation, kind of like creating their own sex toys. Not to mention what some see as animal "cheating"—that is, how some animals seem to secretly have sex with animals who aren't their mates. Is it really a secret? We don't know, of course (given that we can't ask). But the sex appears to be done in private, which makes some researchers think they don't want their "mate" to know. To learn more about the curious sex lives of animals, check out *Sexual Selections: What We Can (and Can't) Learn about Sex from Animals* by Marlene Zuk.

COMMUNICATING FOR BETTER SEX

To have the sex life you crave, you have to go out on a limb. You have to ask for it. At the very least, consider sharing with your partner what it is that you dream of, what makes you aroused, and the kinds of sex dreams you fall asleep thinking about or use during masturbation to become more aroused or to more easily experience orgasm.

This isn't necessarily easy. Many people find it difficult to share their sexual fantasies, especially if they worry that their fantazies are unusual, strange, or possibly "perverted" (I hear that word a lot; however, most of the fantasies people tell me they have are pretty common—things like acting out domination/submission fantasies, having sex with a stranger, having sex with a group of people, and so on).

Having a richer, more interesting sex life also involves listening with compassion and empathy. If your partner asks to try something new, try to respond with kindness even if—perhaps *especially* if—it is something you're not interested in doing. It may have taken your partner significant courage to share their idea with you (even if they seem confident or bold).

If your partner asks you to do something you feel unsure about, try saying something like, "I hadn't thought of that before,—let me take some time to think about it." This gives you a chance to mull over their request on your own time and to learn more about what your partner wants to do. For example, if your partner wants to watch porn together and you're not experienced watching porn, it gives you a chance to seek out types of porn that you might find appealing. If your partner wants to try anal sex, it gives you a chance to read about it first, to learn about STI risk, lubricant use, comfortable anal sex positions, and more. You can also ask your partner for more information or to explore the idea with you before you consider trying it. You can read a book together or talk about your ideas over dinner or a bottle of wine.

On the other hand, if your partner shares a sex idea that you're excited about or open to, that's great. When you share your excitement with your partner, he or she may feel proud that they shared their sex idea or fantasy with you, and reassured that you're into the idea. Again, if you have questions or curiosities, you two still have the chance to learn more together before taking the plunge. Just because you're both game for trying something new doesn't mean you have to try it right away. There's always time to read a book, buy some lube, charge your batteries, buy a new sex toy, or do whatever you need to do to prepare for your sexploration.

— Making It Easy —

73. What to do if . . . your partner wants to do something sexual that you don't want to do

Define something you "don't want to do." If the thing your partner wants to do horrifies you or would make you feel very uncomfortable, remember that you never need to do anything sexual that you don't want to do. You can say no. If you have a partner who doesn't let you say no or who abuses you, talk to someone you trust and get help, such as from a health care provider, counselor, or domestic abuse organization.

If, on the other hand, your partner wants to do something that doesn't particularly excite you but doesn't horrify you either, ask yourself if you might be willing to play with them in this way. Sex is, after all, an adult form of play. When I was growing up, I liked to play with Barbie dolls and my sister liked to play with My Little Pony dolls. Neither of us were big fans of the others' games but we only had each other and no other siblings. We were, if you will, in an "exclusive, non-sexual, but monogamous sibling relationship"—in other words, two sisters with no other brothers or sisters. How did we make this work? Well, we certainly didn't only play games that we both liked playing, games like Operation and Monopoly. Rather, we made deals. We played each other's favorite games even though they weren't our own favorites. I played My Little Pony even though it wasn't my favorite. And a few minutes into playing with her, I often found myself having fun. My sister would play Barbie with me, dressing them up and combing their hair and taking them to their fancy activities. And though she probably didn't admit it growing up, I think she had fun doing it more often than not.

Sex isn't much different. You just have to be a willing, giving, open-minded partner who cares enough about the person they're with that they're willing to do things that wouldn't normally top their "favorite sex things" list. If your partner likes to 69 and you don't, would it bother you that much to put their genitals in your mouth while they lick or kiss yours? Probably not—especially if it meant that your partner was willing to do the thing you enjoy (Make out for an hour? Have sex in the car? Let you use a vibrator on him or her? You get the picture). This is especially important if you are in a monogamous relationship and only have each other to play with, much as my sister and I only had one another. Try to be open-minded with your partner. After all, it's not terribly fair to refuse to go down on your partner if you're not willing to ever let them receive oral sex from anyone else and they are someone who loves oral sex. If you're going to nix any possibility of you two being with others, then at least be open-minded and playful with each other to the extent you can be. You still get to veto anything you absolutely don't want to do; but do try to imagine a greater number of sexual possibilities. Who knows? You might end up liking something new yourself.

74. What to do if . . . your partner wants you to watch porn together

If your partner wants to watch porn with you and you're into porn yourself, great! Talk about your interests and try to find one that interests both of you enough to want to watch it together. Then talk about how you want to do it. Will it be a straight-up movie night with popcorn while you watch porn and laugh about it together (some people see porn as a form of comedy)? Does one of you want to use it as "background" to your own sexual sharing? Or do you want to watch it for inspiration and then try out some of the sex positions or sex acts you observe? Talk about it first, then put it into play.

If you're not into porn, ask yourself if you would be willing to give it a try with your partner. Are there certain conditions that might make it more palatable? As the partner who's not-so-into-it, you have a good deal of negotiating power. Use it. You could agree to watch porn together under the condition that you get to pick the porn movie or that you get to pick three movies or online video clips. Having a choice gives you more freedom to move on to the next one if the first one is unappealing. Remember, too, that you can push "pause" or end the video any time you want. If you try it and don't like it, that's OK. Ask your partner what he or she likes about porn, and why he or she wants to watch it together. Hearing your partner's perspective might help you to see porn through their eyes and may end up inspiring you to like something you never knew you'd be into.

75. What to do if . . . you worry that your partner watches too much porn

Start with a reality check. Ask yourself what you mean by "too much porn." The vast majority of men in countries where porn is readily available—whether in the form of magazines, books, films, videos, or online clips—have watched porn. Most women in the US have seen porn too, although it's less clear how many women who have watched porn have done so in order to feel aroused or make their orgasm easier versus to please their partner.

Some people feel that watching any amount of porn is simply "too much porn," and if you and your partner are in agreement that porn shouldn't be part of your private or shared sexual lives, then you may have a case for asking him or her to nix it. Better yet, though, check in and see if you both still feel that way. People change, as do their beliefs about sex (and sometimes porn). Make sure that you're not pressuring or coercing your partner to be someone they're not or to feel bad or ashamed about their sexuality.

Other people have a sense that porn is a common part of many people's sexual lives and isn't necessarily a problem. Many men I've spoken with have told me that watching porn is a very different experience to them from sex with a real live human partner. They often cannot understand why their girlfriends or wives get upset that they watch porn, particularly as it's some-thing that most men do, or have done, and they often grew up watching porn. A number of my male college students report having watched porn since they were eight, ten, or twelve years old, often skirting around their parents' restrictions and parental-control computer programs in order to find porn and keep it hidden on the family computer. If you think your partner's porn use might be more frequent than you'd like but not a prob-lem, try to reassure yourself of two things: (1) that your partner's porn use isn't necessarily a bad thing if it's not hurting your relationship and (2) that it's OK to feel bothered by it, and that expressing this to your partner in a gentle way that doesn't involve blame or criticism can be healthy. It's OK to say something like, "I want you to know how I feel about your watching porn because I think it would help if we could talk about my feelings and if you could help me to understand yours."

In rare cases, someone may feel as though their or their partner's sex-ual behavior, including their porn watching, is truly out of control. I know of several men who would seek out illegal porn during times in their lives when they were feeling stressed out because of work or family issues, and in some instances this led to the men being arrested. I know of other instances in which men and women have watched porn so frequently that they used it to avoid having sex with or being intimate with their partner. That can certainly be a problem. It doesn't necessarily mean that the person has a "porn addiction" (many sex researchers, including me, are uncomfortable using the term "porn addiction"). However, it may mean that they could use help learning to control their behavior and deal with their relationship issues head-on rather than hide from them. People who have difficulty in these areas can often benefit from seeing a counselor or therapist—preferably one (in my opinion) who doesn't subscribe to the whole "porn addiction" model.

The bottom line is this: ask yourself whether your partner's porn use is truly too much. If not, try to adjust your perspective and maybe even join in on occasion to see how you might be able to incorporate porn into your shared sexual life. And if the porn use is a problem, seek help together from a counselor or therapist.

76. What to do if . . . you wonder if your partner has a "sex addiction"

As you may guess from my response to the porn addiction issue above, I'm not a fan of the "addiction model" as it relates to sex. I don't buy into the idea that people are generally addicted to porn or sex the way they may be to alcohol or drugs. That doesn't mean that some people don't have great difficulty regulating their sexual behavior and their impulses. I know of a number of people (mostly men, but some women) who have found it very difficult to control their sexual behavior. Some of these individuals have risked their relationships or even gotten arrested for breaking into friends' houses to go through their underwear drawers and masturbate. Another person I'm aware of used to sneak into a firehouse to try on firemen's clothes for sexual gratification. Others have masturbated so often or with such force that they have unintentionally rubbed their genital skin raw, and then done it again the next week. Some other people have risked acquiring HIV, or risked their relationship or marriage, by having unprotected sex with people whose names they didn't know, and they couldn't stop doing so no matter how hard they tried.

I hope that by reading about these instances you get a sense of the types of sexual behaviors that those of us who work in the fields of sex research or therapy often find "problematic." They tend to involve people putting themselves in extreme situations and wanting to change their behavior, but feeling challenged by a sense that they are unable to control it. This is far different from the cases of "sex addiction" I often get asked about in my work. Too often, women have told me that they worry their partner is "addicted to sex" because he wants to have sex with them every day or because he masturbates three times a week. Wanting to have sex with one's partner every day may be ambitious, but it's unlikely to be an addiction. And masturbating several times a week is common among men; some women masturbate frequently too (though more often when they're younger and more often when they're not regularly having sex with a partner).

If you and your partner have different sex drives or sexual preferences or interests, that's one thing—and it's not likely that they have an "addiction" just because they want more sex or kinkier sex than you do. If your partner finds it difficult to control their sexual behavior—and particularly if you or your partner finds that sex is getting in the way of your relationship, family life, or employment or that they or you are running the risk of getting arrested—you may find it helpful to speak with a sex therapist.

77. What to do if . . . you want to try fisting

Based on limited scientific data, fisting appears to be a relatively uncommon sexual behavior; however, it's certainly one that many men and women try, enjoy—and have questions about. There are several important things to know if you and your partner are considering trying fisting. First, you should read a great deal about vaginal or anal fisting before engaging in either one. Two options include *A Hand in the Bush: The Fine Art of Vaginal Fisting* (Greenery Press) and *Susie Sexpert's Lesbian Sex World* (Bright Stuff). Second, contrary to what many people guess, fisting has nothing to do with inserting a full fist into a person's vagina or anus. That would hurt most people—badly. Rather, fisting typically involves starting slowly with inserting one lubricated finger, then two lubricated fingers, and so on. As a couple becomes more familiar with each other, and more experienced, they may decide to try inserting an entire well-lubricated and often glove-covered hand into the vagina or anus (the glove being a disposable latex glove or similar, not a winter glove!). The hand is *not* made into a fist first; instead, people tend to smoosh their fingers together in a shape almost like a bird's beak so as to make the size of their hand as small and comfortable as possible for insertion. See? It gets complicated. That's why I suggest reading a great deal about fisting before trying it; that way, you have a higher chance of having a safer and more pleasurable experience than one that hurts. Fisting is also one of those sexual behaviors that are best done with someone you know very well, trust completely, and feel you can say anything to—including "Stop," "More," or "Be gentle."

78. What to do if . . . you lose the key to your fuzzy handcuffs while they're on

Hopefully you're using handcuffs with a safety release, such as a button or latch on the side that can be pressed for a quick release without needing a key. If not—and if you or your partner is stuck inside the handcuffs—do not attempt to cut them loose on your own. Instead, go to the emergency room for assistance or call the paramedics if you cannot safely get to the emergency room on your own. You may be able to call your local police department for help as well.

79. What to do if . . . you can't stop fantasizing about other people during sex

In a 2007 study, researchers at the University of Vermont surveyed 349 women and men ages eighteen to seventy who were in relationships. They found that in the previous two months alone, 98 percent of men and 80 percent of women had had a sexual fantasy involving another person.[6] This tells me that in many ways we are similar to other animals in that sexual desire and arousal are natural impulses. Just because a person's own values or culture puts sex into a neat little box—one that says we should only have sexual thoughts, feelings, or fantasies about a monogamous-relationship partner—it doesn't mean that's how our minds and bodies work. It is common to have sexual fantasies about people other than one's relationship partner. As the old saying goes, "It doesn't matter where your partner gets their appetite, as long as they eat at home" (at least that's the case for people in monogamous relationships).

That said, if you find that you are unable to become aroused by thinking about your partner, you might want to examine the issue further. Some women and men feel that they "get through sex" by thinking about other people, which may make them feel guilty or sad that thinking about their partner doesn't do much for them. Some people are able to redirect their thoughts to their sexual partner and become aroused by being with their partner. You may even find that mindfulness techniques (in which you focus on how sex with your partner looks, feels, smells, and tastes) help you enhance your arousal with your partner, just as they've helped women in some research studies.

Reading *Passionate Marriage* (mentioned elsewhere in this book) may help as well; one of the first examples in the book involves a woman who almost always fantasizes about someone else and, through counseling and greater emotional intimacy with her husband, finds ways to involve him in her fantasy life and focus on the present moment when she has sex with him. Finally, sex therapy may be a helpful option for women and couples experiencing this situation.

80. What to do if . . . you're straight but dream about having sex with other women

Dreams don't always accurately reflect who we are in waking life. Women and men of all sexual orientations may have dreams about having sex with women, men, or groups of women and men. Two gay male friends have separately told me that—much to their own surprise—they had dreamed about having sex with me. At different points in my life, I've had sex dreams about men and women I was definitely not into. The first time I remember it happening is when I had a sex dream about a guy from my high school whom I most certainly did not like "in that way." Seeing him the next day at school, I felt so embarrassed, as if he would somehow telepathically know about the explicit dream I had about him.

People's sex dreams are all over the map. Straight women who are entirely into men sometimes have sex dreams about women. Also, lesbians who are entirely into women sometimes have sex dreams that involve men. We don't understand much about people's dreams and why we dream about the things that we do. Take your dreams with a grain of salt.

If you're only into men and wake up wondering what your sex dreams involving other women are about, you might ask yourself if there's a woman in your life you're interested in. If not, shrug it off and go on with your day. If you are sexually interested in a woman, you might spend some time thinking about this and what it is that's holding you back from pursuing your interest in her. Throughout life it's likely that you'll have a number of sex dreams and that a good number may involve sexual experiences you would never be interested in pursuing in waking life. They're only dreams.

81. What to do if . . . you're in a relationship and want to bring someone in for a threesome

Many women and men ask me for advice about threesomes. For many women, it's one thing to ask your best girlfriend for advice on choosing a lubricant and an entirely different matter to ask about threesomes (which are more taboo in our culture). Asking a stranger (like me) for advice on sensitive topics can feel easier than asking a friend.

Most people who ask me about threesomes want to know if they should have one or if having a threesome will ruin their relationship. I can't answer that for anyone. Some people find that having a threesome adds to their relationship and makes sex, and their intimate connection, more exciting. I know some straight, gay, and lesbian couples who enjoy involving others in their sex lives. One gay couple I know has a regular threesome partner who joins them for sex a few times a year, and it seems to work well for all involved. A straight couple I know enjoys going to sex clubs when they travel. And a heteroflexible woman I know (she feels mostly straight with the occasional interest in women) has joined straight couples in their sex play and, in other instances, has sought out a female partner to join her and her boyfriend.

For other people, having a threesome poses serious problems. I know of one woman who had a threesome with her husband and a male friend and then became pregnant and didn't know whose baby it was, prompting her and her husband to choose to terminate the pregnancy (get an abortion). And I know of a number of threesomes that have ended up with one person transmitting an STI to one of their sex partners. There are also many instances in which people have threesomes for the wrong reasons, like trying to keep their partner interested in them, or trying to fix a relationship that is already tanking beyond anyone's ability to save it. Having a threesome as a last-ditch effort to save a relationship is not a great idea, in my opinion, and often results in heartbreak or fighting.

If, on the other hand, you're having a threesome to enhance an already stable and healthy relationship, it may go just fine. My advice, though, is to talk about it with your partner ahead of time and figure out your "rules" and boundaries. You might want to talk about

- **Who you'll seek out as your third partner.** Will it be a woman or a man? A close friend, an ex, or a stranger you connect with online? Someone you meet at a sex club or a neighborhood bar? These are different kinds of people with different pros and cons you should consider before settling on someone to approach about joining you two for sex.

- **No surprises.** This is an important rule to threesomes; you need to respect your partner's right to privacy and how their sex life happens. Even if you've agreed you want to have a threesome, it's not OK to post pictures of your partner on CraigsList or Adult Friend Finder or a swinging app or site unless your partner has agreed to it. Pictures on the Internet have a way of making their way into the wrong hands, so be respectful about what you put into the world in your quest for finding a threesome partner.

- **Precautions you'll take for safer sex.** Particularly if you two have been in a monogamous relationship, it may have been a while since you've thought about safer sex, let alone had to practice it. If it's been some time, you'll want to buy condoms (or make sure that the condoms you have on hand haven't yet hit their expiration date) and any new sex toys you'd like to use with the third person. For hygiene and safer sex reasons, it's not wise to use your sex toys with a new person whose STI and health history you don't know. You may also want to communicate with the third person about their STI history and testing. And if you haven't had an HPV vaccine, ask your health care provider if you and your partner are good candidates for it.

• **Types of sex you can have—or should avoid.** For some couples, having a threesome is a no-holds-barred, exploratory experience in which they can do whatever they want with each other as long as everyone consents to it. Others talk in advance about what is and is not OK with them (Is kissing OK? Oral sex? Vaginal sex? etc.). Decide on your rules and stick to them.

• **The combinations that work well for you.** There's no right way to do it and there is a lot of variation. In threesomes involving two women and one man, some women want to have sex with the second female partner but don't want their boyfriends or husbands to be sexual with her. Other women want to watch their male partners receive oral sex from the other woman, or else they both want to take turns receiving vaginal sex from him (using a different condom for each woman). In threesomes involving a woman and two men, some women want to be penetrated by both men at the same time (such as oral sex and vaginal sex or vaginal sex and anal sex). Other women are turned on by seeing their male partner being sexual with the second man.

• **What will happen afterward.** You might want to take the approach that you're all viewing this as a one-time experience and can talk later on about what went well, what didn't go as hoped for, and whether you want to try it again together. But there are other things to decide: Will this person sleep over at your house or go home afterward? Or will you all meet at a hotel for sex and then go your separate ways?

What about post-threesome communication: is it OK in your relationship if you and/or your partner become Facebook friends with the third person? Or start to text? Or should all communication end when the threesome is over?

There are numerous ways to have a threesome and talking about it ahead of time will give you, your partner, and your threesome partner a better chance of having a sexual experience that is pleasurable for all.

82. What to do if . . . you're both curious about him giving you a facial

In sex-speak, a facial is when a man ejaculates on his partner's face: it's not exactly an aromatherapy salon facial. Facials are common in porn, which has resulted in many men and women thinking that they are common in real life (outside the porn world). I know of no scientific data that can speak to how rare or how common it is. My guess is that many people have tried them but few people engage in them with any regularity. However, I get enough questions about facials from women and men that I suspect more people could use helpful information on the topic, so here we are.

Some women find the idea of a facial to be highly offensive, disgusting, and/or a negative sign of how porn influences people's sex lives. Others feel neutral about the idea; they're not particularly into it but are open to the idea if it's something their partner wants to do. Then there are women who feel turned on by the idea of their male partner coming on their face (or of their female partner coming on their face, if she is someone who experiences female ejaculation). A good friend once overheard his roommate's girlfriend begging him to come on her face. If you're thinking of trying a facial, here are some tips to make it a better experience:

• **Consider cleanup.** Some women and their partners take their facials into the shower for easier cleanup. Others keep a towel or wet sex wipes nearby.

• **Think about STIs ahead of time.** If you're not sure about your partner's STI status, think twice before asking for or agreeing to a facial. If he has an STI and his semen accidentally gets into your eye or your mouth, he could transmit it to you. If he has pubic lice (crabs) and his pubic hair get too close to your eyelashes, the lice may jump ship from his pubic hair to your eyelashes.

• **Use the hand shield maneuver.** Take steps to protect your eyes from your partner's semen, which can sting and burn if it accidentally gets into your eye—even just a little bit. Ask him to aim elsewhere (such as your cheeks or close to your mouth) and hold your hand in front of your eyes to protect them from flying semen.

If you accidentally get semen in your eye, trying splashing your eye with room-temperature water to help get the semen out or dilute it. If you wear contacts, you may be more comfortable removing your contacts and wearing your glasses for a day or two until any irritation subsides. If your eyes hurt or become very red or pink, or if you simply have questions about your eye health or whether you've gotten an STI from your partner, you may want to check in with an ophthalmologist (a doctor who specializes in eye health).

83. What to do if . . . he wants to experiment with other men

Perhaps you've been at a party where guys egg women on to make out with each other, or maybe you've been at a bar and watched as two women make out with each other to get free drinks from a bartender. Yet there aren't really any male equivalents of these scenes. For some reason, women are often encouraged to explore sexually with one another and men aren't. However, some men—like some women—are curious about being sexual with each other. In our national sex study, we found that a number of men reported having had sex with other men but didn't identify as gay or bisexual. This echoes the findings of other research that has found these gray areas of sexual identify and behavior.

If you've always known that your partner identifies as bisexual, or if you're aware of instances in his past that have involved him having sex with men, his desire to have sex with other men may not surprise you. If you've always thought of your boyfriend or husband as straight, however, you might not be sure what to think if he says he'd like to try being sexual with another man. And frankly, there's no way to know where things are headed when a man wants to have sex with another man.

It's possible that your boyfriend or husband is gay, is mostly or entirely attracted to men, and tried to make a go of it as a straight guy. His exploration may be a way to keep one foot on safe ground by staying with you as he checks out what it's like to explore his previously unexplored desire for men. It's also possible that your boyfriend or husband is very much into women (including you) and also happens to be sexually interested in or turned on by men. This doesn't have to be a threat to your relationship. The question is what to do about it.

If you and your partner are in a monogamous relationship, you need to talk and decide whether you want to continue being monogamous or whether you're comfortable opening it up so that he can explore his interest in men, either on his own or as part of a threesome with you. If you want to stay monogamous and he doesn't because he wants to explore with men, perhaps the time has come to end the relationship. If you two want to stay together and keep it monogamous, you may find a way to incorporate his sexual fantasies into your own sex life. Some couples are very inventive when it comes to dirty talk and sharing sexual fantasies with one another; you may be able to "talk" your way through a situation that involves the two of you going out to a bar and meeting a man and bringing him home to have sex with both of you or with your boyfriend/husband. Or you might want to watch gay porn together. There are several ways to make this work, depending on your shared wishes. Another option is to go to a sex club together and find some way to incorporate his desires as well as whatever your own desires may be. For example, your boyfriend/husband might feel turned on by seeing other naked men in the room even though you've decided that he will have sex only with you. Or, if you're both into it, you may be able to find a man there to have sex with the both of you or another couple that would be open to playing with you two in mutually pleasurable ways.

84. What to do if . . . your partner wants you to gain lots of weight as a turn-on

A very small percentage of people are into what's called "feederism," which is a sexual preference that involves sexual arousal or gratification from the process of gaining body fat. There are feeders (the person who wants their partner to gain weight) and feedees (also called gainers, the individual who gains weight to sexually turn on or please their partner). This is an aspect of human sexuality that is not well understood and hasn't been studied much. However, some sex therapists I know are concerned that feederism involves—at least in some cases—people manipulating others into doing something (sometimes gaining a very large amount of weight) that may be physically unhealthy for them, and that this may be done in an emotionally abusive way. Of course, that doesn't mean it's never done in a consensual and healthy way; it's certainly the case that the people sex therapists see are often individuals who feel troubled by their sex lives rather than people who feel healthy and happy about the way they experience their sex lives.

My take is this: if your partner wants you to do something for your sex life that you don't feel good about, don't do it. If a sexual partner asks you to do something that feels risky or unhealthy, or you have questions about it, talk with your health care provider or a counselor. Sometimes people pressure their sexual partners to gain weight, lose weight, start smoking, or have sex with people they don't know well. If you're feeling pressured, manipulated, or coerced into doing something that you don't feel comfortable with, seek help from a friend, counselor, therapist, or another trusted person.

All that said, if your sexual practices feel "outside the norm" but you enjoy and feel good about them, that, too, can be healthy. It can feel good to know that one's sex life is what one wants—even if (and sometimes especially if) it's unconventional.

85. What to do if . . . you run into someone you know at a sex club

Some people don't want to be seen at a sex club and go to great lengths to avoid it, such as only going to sex clubs when they travel away from home. Others go to local sex spaces and aren't concerned about seeing friends, coworkers, or neighbors. There are many ways to look at the issue of running into others.

You might decide that it's OK. Even if you're embarrassed to have been seen at a sex club, the fact is that you saw this other person there too. You're in the same boat. Nod your head, say hi, and move on.

On the plus side, if you've long found this other person attractive, you've now perhaps had the chance to see them in fewer clothes or even naked. Not a bad night! Maybe you'll even get a chance to be sexual together, now that you both know that the other one is into sexual exploration within a sex club environment. Once you're outside the club, keep your acquaintance's confidence. It's not anyone else's business whom you saw here. If you're worried about that person sharing your private information with others, ask him or her to please keep your whereabouts between the two of you.

Finally, if you feel very anxious about people knowing you're at a sex club, it might be the case that going to a sex club is not for you. Some politicians would have perhaps been better off if they had made different sexual choices. If your relationship or job would be in serious jeopardy if people learned you were at a sex club, you may want to spend time thinking about whether there are ways to explore your sexual desires in a more private way, such as at a sex club that's known for greater confidentiality. (Clubs vary greatly in this regard; some can be attended by anyone who walks in and pays a fee, whereas others require an application, essay writing, photos, an interview, and possibly a probationary period. Choose wisely.)

86. What to do if . . . you want to make a homemade sex tape

Again, your choices will in part be guided by how you feel about the possibility of your tape ever accidentally finding its way into the public. If the idea absolutely terrifies you, either don't make a sex tape or film it on your camera, watch it together right after making it, and then delete it immediately.

If you and your partner aren't as worried about the tape ever being made public, then you may feel comfortable taking more chances. You may feel comfortable shooting the video in a way that shows your faces. You may also feel comfortable with the idea that both you and your partner get to keep a copy of your homemade sex tape. You may even like the idea of uploading it to an amateur porn site and sharing it with the world. Only do this if you both are in 100 percent agreement that you want to do this, if you are certain that uploading your video to a site is in compliance with relevant laws, and if you are both sober when making this decision.

A few final tips: Watching oneself on film is significantly different from having sex in the moment. Try to choose light that is flattering enough for the both of you and still bright enough for taping. Some people film using a tripod, whereas others prefer to pass the camera back and forth between each other, taking turns at being the "director."

Sex Smarts Quiz

1. Which group of Americans are among the best condom users—at least when it comes to using condoms with casual sex partners?
    a. Teenagers
    b. Men in their twenties
    c. Women in their thirties
    d. Women in their forties
2. As many as _____ percent of men and women in some age groups have had anal sex.
    a. 5 to 10 percent
    b. 15 to 20 percent
    c. 20 to 25 percent
    d. 40 to 45 percent
3. Which STI can be easily transmitted from a person's pubic hair to their partner's eyelashes if these parts get too close?
    a. Herpes
    b. HPV
    c. Pubic lice
    d. Trich

Answers
    1. a
    2. d
    3. c

Chapter 9

When Life Gets in the Way: How to Manage Sex in the Midst of Dogs, Cats, Kids, Injuries, Roommates, and Neighbors

Sex can feel challenging enough all on its own, yet it doesn't exist in a vacuum. Sex is one part of a larger experience of life that may include pets, children, a person's career, health issues, pregnancies, and roommates or neighbors with whom we share space. A person's sex life is never just about sex; it's a balancing act. Just when you think you have one part down (for example, getting your desire back after a dry spell), it may be that your partner gets sick, throwing everything out of whack again. Or maybe you adopt a puppy whose needs for early-morning walks spell the end of your morning sex. It happens. And here in this chapter, you'll find tips to help you to navigate these tricky intersections of sex, life, and love.

DISTRACTING, ISN'T IT?

It's good to be a "thinking" person—but this isn't always the case during sex. Many women and men could benefit from learning to relax, let go, and enjoy the emotional and physical experiences of sex. Decades ago, pioneering sex researchers William Masters and Virginia Johnson theorized that "spectatoring"—a process that involves people observing themselves from a third-party perspective—plays a part in people's sexual difficulties. This is the idea that, instead of surrendering himself to pleasure, a man may think to himself *Come on, last longer, last longer, you can do it* or a woman may think to herself *"Ugh, why can't I have an orgasm? Why is this so diffi-cult for me?"*

Spectatoring interrupts many people's sexual experiences with worries and criticisms. A 2006 study published in the *Journal of Sex Research* found that women were more prone to these types of cognitive distractions (sci-ence-speak for the thoughts we'd all love to make go away sometimes) than men.[1] In particular, we women seem more vulnerable to worrying about how our bodies look while we're having sex, though certainly some men are vulnerable to body image concerns too. When I first started teaching human sexuality classes to college students, I was struck by how many col-lege-aged men would say that they preferred to have sex in the missionary position because they felt it made their chest and arms look stronger.

Thoughts that distract people during sex can come in many forms. They can be the spectatoring kind that are about a person's performance. The 2006 study just mentioned found that women and men are similarly prone to experiencing distracting thoughts related to performance; men often worry about their erections and lasting longer. Women often worry about orgasms.

But performance and body image aren't the only types of thoughts or worries that creep into the minds of women and men during sex. Perhaps, like many people, you have been in the middle of having sex when suddenly a thought pops into your mind and you

- Wonder if you turned the stove off
- Think about laundry that needs to get done
- Remember that you have an exam to take or a presentation due the next day
- Think how your wedding is weeks away and you still don't have all the RSVPs returned to you
- Are distracted by your dog's stares or your cat scratching at the door
- Try to remember if you missed any birth control pills lately
- Wonder if you locked the bedroom door, in case your child gets up and wanders in
- Wonder if the condom is still on

• Hope that this time you will be able to become pregnant

I've been in several of these situations; most of us have. As much as many of us would love to throw caution to the wind and enjoy sex, worrying about "life" and its many details is common. In a recent study, published in 2011 in *Archives of Sexual Behavior*, researchers at the University of Central Florida found that many people worried about their STI risk when they had sex (men more so than women).[2] They also found that heterosexual women and gay men more often worried about their bodies and appearance during sex. Even more so than heterosexual women, lesbian women tended to focus on their physical performance (such as whether they were satisfying their partner or whether their partner was having an orgasm).

Some research has found that mindfulness techniques can help enhance women's arousal and orgasm.[3-4] They can certainly help people to focus on living in the present. If you find yourself prone to cognitive distractions (whether about performance, body image, laundry, or anything else), try to breathe deeply during sex and redirect your thoughts to how it feels to touch your partner, breathe in the scent of his or her skin and hair, or feel the sheets against your skin. There may also be steps you can take to have a more relaxing experience of sex. Before heading to bed, you might go through your to-do list to see if you've checked off the most important tasks. And if you're headed out on a date that might include sex, be sure to pack condoms, lubricant, and anything else that will create a safer, more enjoyable space for pleasure.

SEX AND YOUR HEALTH

Thinking distracting thoughts isn't the only possible sex interruption. Health problems can change the way an individual or a coupleexperiences sex too. Most of us will experience significant health issues at one time or another. And if it doesn't happen to us, something serious enough to impact sex may happen to our partner (which ultimately affects both partners).

A number of health issues can affect a person's sex life including diabetes, heart problems, cancer and cancer treatments, a sprained or broken knee, having hip replacement surgery, and so on. Sex can even be impacted by allergies, a bad cold, a week spent with the flu, or a case of bronchitis or pneumonia.

If you're experiencing an ongoing or difficult health issue, please talk with your health care provider for an accurate diagnosis, treatment options, and steps to take to improve your quality of life—as well as information about managing your sex life. Try to think about your health in big-picture terms. If your health issue (for example, knee pain) gets in the way of your ability to get a good night's sleep, then part of the way to improve your sex life will start with asking your health care provider what you can do to manage your knee pain in a way that also allows you to experience restful sleep. After all, if you're in pain or grumpy from bad sleep, you probably won't be in the best position to create great sex. Once you get issues like pain and sleep under control, then you can turn your attention to more specific sex issues, such as asking your health care provider or physical therapist about sex positions that might work particularly well for people who have knee problems like yours.

Sometimes doctors and physical therapists don't have answers to questions about sex; often they received little information about sexual behavior during their professional training. Some people who have significant health issues find it helpful to connect with online or in-person patient support groups and ask one another these kinds of questions. However, if someone in one of these support groups suggests trying something that you have reservations about, it is always wise to ask your health care provider for their thoughts on how safe this suggestion may be. Sometimes such suggestions are brilliant bursts of creativity, and sharing them with your health care provider may mean that they learn from them and can pass them along to other patients. Other times, such suggestions can be misguided at best and dangerous at worst, which is why it's wise to bring health-related questions back to your health care provider.

Post-Pet Sex

In addition to being distracted by health issues (such as pain and discomfort), some people are distracted by their pets during sex. That's right: their pets. According to the 2007 *US Pet Ownership & Demographics Sourcebook*, in the US there are more than 43 million households that have a dog and more than 37 million households with a cat.[5] Although I grew up with pets (both dogs and cats), it was a long time before I adopted one as an adult. For years, I would listen in amazement to friends, students, and readers talk about how their pets influenced their sex lives. I have one friend, for example, who would try to shut her cats out of her bedroom during sex only to find them scratching and meowing at her door. Another friend avoided having sex in her apartment because she worried about her cats—who she felt were like her "babies"—seeing her in such "compromising" sex positions. Someone else told me she felt like her nosy dog was always interrupting sex with her boyfriend. And then there's the opening (hilarious) scene of the mockumentary *Best in Show*, in which a couple visits a pet therapist to discuss how their dog has possibly been affected by witnessing them have certain types of sex.

After years of listening to these stories, and then adopting our own shelter dog, I decided it was time to study the topic. In a study I conducted at Indiana University, I surveyed close to two thousand men and women about how their sex lives were affected by their dogs and cats, if at all. People had all sorts of stories to tell, including being distracted by their pets during sex (such as worrying that their pets would run across the bed during sex, or by hearing their pet at the door). Others didn't feel too bothered and felt that it all worked out pretty well in their homes, with pets and humans having a happy coexistence. Consider these excerpts from participants' stories (their names have been changed):

> *The cats seem to be very interested in the smells after sex, but sort of scared off by the activity itself. It hasn't been an issue. One of the cats loves to snuggle against me when I masturbate. That doesn't bother me. The other cat was too*

interested in the movements of my hand under the blankets, so I carefully arrange the blankets, or even hide under a pillow so she can't see what's going on and pounce.

—Donna, age forty-five

We have a guest room that we designate as our "boom boom" room. When we are about to be intimate, we leave our dog in the master bedroom, with the TV on, and we go to our "boom boom" room and enjoy each other. When we return, he hardly notices that we left.

—Tom, age thirty

The cats don't really interfere too much. We close the door, and they leave us alone. Except for one cat, who gets very upset when we do bondage. She mews and squeaks and shakes her tail—which totally kills the mood. So we kick her out of whatever room we're in.

—Bree, age thirty-three

My dog isn't allowed in the bedroom, so we only have sex in there. We always close the door because, due to previous experience, the dog will look in and make noise. If we are in an area the dog has access to she wants to lick or poke at us and will climb on us. I feel really strange having relations with the dog watching.

—Jamie, age twenty-one

Though pets are certainly not human babies, for many people having a pet feels very much like having a baby that they care for, love, and protect. Perhaps it comes as no surprise, then, that having sex in front of this "baby-like" being can feel strange and like something they want to avoid at all costs. Hence, the idea of "post-pet sex": the sense that there's the way one's sex life happened before getting a dog or cat and the way sex changed afterward. It's not that one is necessarily better or worse, but many pet owners would certainly say that they are different experiences.

In my study, many people described their post-pet sex lives as something of a work in progress. Some women and men wrote about their sex lives being more challenged when their dogs were young puppies and had boundless energy and a need to get up multiple times throughout the night. However, the mellowing that comes with a dog or cat's older age meant fewer sex interruptions for some of the women and men in my study. These individuals also wrote about trying a number of strategies until they hit upon something that worked: Some people distracted their cats with catnip or a windup toy. Some dog owners gave their dog a peanut butter–filled toy before retreating to the bedroom, and others simply shut their pets out of the room. Later on in this chapter, we'll consider several examples of post-pet sex that works.

BETTER BABY-MAKING SEX

About half of pregnancies in the US are unplanned, which means that the other half of pregnancies involve some amount of planning or, dare I say it, "work." For some couples, the work of becoming pregnant is fun. For the first time in a long time—maybe even for the first time in their lives—they get to ditch condoms, birth control, and worries about becoming pregnant. Sex that's free of such stressors can feel uninhibited and exciting. Creating a baby together can feel highly connecting, loving, and even spiritual.

However, pregnancy doesn't happen effortlessly for all couples. According to a report by the Pew Research Center that is based on data from the National Center for Health Statistics and the Census Bureau, in 2008 about 14 percent of births were to women ages thirty-five and older.[6] Many of these pregnancies (as well as a number of pregnancies for women younger than thirty-five) take more planning and often significant efforts involving changes to sex as well as various fertility treatments.

There is no easy way to make baby-making sex perfect in every way, but there are steps couples can take to have a more pleasurable experience. This is important because oftentimes couples feel that baby-making sex feels too planned, mechanical, or devoid of connection. One man once complained to me that he felt more like a machine than a husband or partner to his wife. He felt a great deal of pressure to perform whenever she ovulated. Women, too, experience a range of feelings about baby-making sex. Here are some thoughts that might improve the way you and your partner experience sex in the midst of trying to have a baby:

• **Try to keep some of your sex spontaneous and unplanned.** Try having sex even on days when you're not likely to be ovulating, simply for the sake of fun and enjoyment. If your partner asks if you're ovulating, say something like, "No, I just want you."

• **Express desire for your partner.** Some couples are able to laugh off the fact that baby-making sex can feel unromantic, planned, and mechanical. Others struggle more with this. If you're trying to become pregnant, add as much desire, romance, or lust to the experience as you can. Rather than an "in, out, and done" experience every time, mix in fun quickies in the kitchen, a drawn-out lovemaking session in the bedroom, and plenty of things (like oral sex) that won't result in pregnancy but can be fun just because.

• **Mix up your sex positions.** Although it may be that some sex positions are better for pregnancy than others (most notably, ones like missionary that have gravity on their side), try not to throw every other sex position out the window. If your partner comes very quickly, save the sex positions that are less pregnancy-friendly for the days when you're unlikely to be ovulating. If your partner can last longer before ejaculating, then front-load your sex play with some of your other favorite sex positions before ending in a bang with your preferred baby-making sex position.

• **Keep talking—and laughing.** Remind yourselves why you're going through all this effort—and sometimes less-than-awesome sex. Talk about having babies. Talk about your family. And sometimes, give it a break. Take hikes together and talk about nature, work, your parents, or the early days of dating. And when sex feels like a science experiment or you're bringing out what looks like a turkey baster or your partner has to march off to ejaculate into a cup at some doctor's office, try to laugh, hug, kiss, and make the best of it.

SEX DURING PREGNANCY: TRIMESTER BY TRIMESTER

Sex during pregnancy comes with its own set of rules, many of which medical doctors and health educators make up as they go along, doing the best they can. Because every pregnancy is different, you should always ask your health care provider any questions that you may have about your own pregnancy and personal health. Consider the below to be general thoughts on pregnancy but not the final word; the final word on what you should or shouldn't be doing during pregnancy comes in a conversation between you and your health care provider.

First Trimester

As long as your pregnancy is proceeding in a healthy way, most health care providers will give you the go-ahead when it comes to sex. Many women are told that they can have sex as often as they want during pregnancy. However, not everyone feels up to it. Some women experience morning sickness during pregnancy and may feel like they're going to throw up, or may actually throw up. It's also common for women to feel unusually tired during their first trimester of pregnancy. If you're in your first trimester and are trying to maintain an active sex life with your partner, note whether there are specific times of the day when you feel healthier, more energetic, and more "yourself." Not all women have morning sickness in the morning; some feel sick and tired later in the afternoon. It varies. If there's a time of day that feels easier for you, talk with your partner about this. Let him or her know that you generally feel sick or tired in the morning, afternoon, or evening (whenever that is). If it's unpredictable when you will feel your best, let your partner know that—and ask if you can take the reins on when to initiate sex for a while.

It's also important to note that although some women worry about having sex for fear of miscarrying, miscarriages tend to be caused by chromosomal abnormalities or other problems with the developing fetus—not by sex or other things you or your partner did or didn't do.

Can Pregnant Women Use Vibrators?

This question comes up often in my work, particularly because some of my research at Indiana University is related to vibrator use. To my knowledge, there have been no scientific studies about vibrator use among pregnant women. This means that we don't know whether it is safe for pregnant women to use vibrators. As a result, some vibrators will come with package inserts that say they are not to be used by pregnant women (this is largely for liability reasons, as no one wants to do anything that would be unsafe for a pregnant woman or her baby). In the real world, this is what we know: in one study my research team conducted, we asked women why they started to use vibrators in the first place. A few women said that they started using a vibrator when they were pregnant. In at least one case that I recall, a woman said that she was pregnant and felt that her husband didn't want to have sex with her, so she started using a vibrator. I've also spoken with several colleagues about this issue. A urologist I know said that she didn't know whether vibrator use was safe, and consequently she probably wouldn't recommend vibrator use to her pregnant patients. On the other hand, a gynecologist told me that a number of her patients have told her that they use vibrators and, as long as their pregnancies are healthy enough to have sex, she doesn't advise against it in her practice and hasn't noticed any problems thus far. If you have questions about vibrator use during your pregnancy, please consult your health care provider.

What About Oral and Anal?

Oral sex is generally considered to be safe for most women to engage in while pregnant. However, their partners need to be extra careful not to blow air into the vagina, lest they run the very rare but real risk of causing an air embolism (which would be dangerous for the mother and baby).

As for anal sex, it often isn't recommended during pregnancy. Women who develop pregnancy-related hemorrhoids may find anal sex uncomfortable. The bigger issue, however, involves accidentally spreading bacteria from the anus into the vagina; during pregnancy, the name of the game is keeping the vagina free of harmful bacteria and infections. Speaking of which, if you are pregnant and having sex with someone other than a monogamous, STI-free partner, consider using condoms to reduce the risk of STI transmission.

Second Trimester

During the second trimester of pregnancy, blood flow increases to women's breasts and genitals. This results in many women feeling strong sexual desire. One woman I know—let's call her Marcy (it's not her real name)—said that she wanted to have sex nearly every day during her second trimester of pregnancy. She had felt tired and sick during her first trimester and wondered how long she would go on feeling that way. Then the second trimester came along and Marcy felt different: her body seemed to have adjusted to the hormonal changes that, in the first trimester, had thrown her for a loop. Now she felt more rested, energetic, excited about her growing "baby bump"—and very excited about having sex. Marcy's husband was pretty excited about it too, though she didn't always wait for him; she engaged in plenty of masturbation as well as sex with him.

Some research has found that women's sexual satisfaction increases during the second trimester, perhaps because women are more likely to feel energetic and aroused (horny) and to have adjusted to their changing bodies.[7] Other research has found that women and their partners experience less sexual desire, less sexual satisfaction, and less frequent sex with each trimester of pregnancy.[8] Again, every pregnancy is different—as is every relationship. It can be difficult not to compare oneself with other women and their relationships, but no matter your experience, know that you're not alone. If your sex drive is in overdrive and your partner is struggling to keep up with you, there are other women like you. And if you're exhausted or not into sex, there are other women out there going through that too.

Third Trimester

Most research about pregnancy and sexuality tends to find that women have less sexual desire during their third trimester of pregnancy and also less frequent sex with their partners. Men tend to feel less sexual desire during this phase as well, perhaps particularly if they worry about hurting the baby or if they see very obviously pregnant-looking women as nonsexual rather than their sexy girlfriends or wives. Some people are more turned on than ever during their partner's third trimester—especially, it seems, if their desire is fueled by feelings of closeness, intimacy, and joy at becoming parents.

For a number of men and women, the joys of being so close to having a baby together inspire greater sexual closeness. And of course it's not all about sex: a 2011 study published in the *Archives of Sexual Behavior* examined the sexual lives and relationships of 361 pregnant and nonpregnant women. In this study, the researchers found that nonpregnant women reported higher levels of sexual desire and intimacy compared to pregnant women (no surprise there).[9] However, pregnant women indicated greater levels of commitment to, and love for, their partner than nonpregnant women. These researchers also followed twenty-five women throughout their pregnancy and found that, compared to the first trimester, women in their third trimester reported significant changes to their sexual and intimate lives. Their relationship quality hadn't really changed; however, they felt less sexual enjoyment and felt less loved by their partner. To me, this underscores the need for partners to keep talking and finding not only new ways to have sex, but also new ways to express love and affection for each other.

That's not to downplay the sex changes that can and do come with the third trimester: With a growing baby bump, sex often changes significantly. Many couples find certain sex positions very difficult to experience. In some positions (like woman on top), a woman's belly may weigh heavily on her partner—though not all partners are bothered by this. Other sex positions may feel uncomfortable for the woman, particularly if the baby is pressing on her bladder or if her back aches or she experiences other types of discomfort. Couples also sometimes struggle to get close enough to each other during sex. Lying side by side is sometimes a preferred third-trimester position, as it allows closeness but also provides support for the stomach. Some women also find rear entry on all fours (doggie style) to be comfortable and pleasurable.

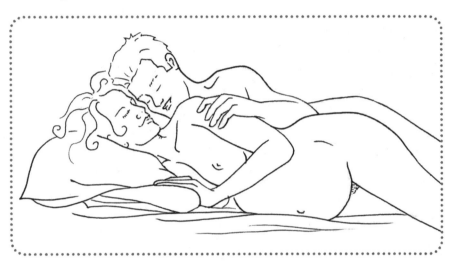

Having sex in a spooning position can be one of the more comfortable sex positions during the third trimester of pregnancy.

Finally, you may have heard the old wives' tale that when you're ready to go into labor, sex may nudge things along. Part of the theory behind this idea rests on the idea that a woman's orgasms—which involve uterine contractions—might encourage labor contractions to begin. Orgasm also involves the release of oxytocin, which can stimulate uterine contractions. I've heard other colleagues who are obstetricians suggest that men's semen, which contains prostaglandins, may help trigger labor (prostaglandins are hormones that are used to help induce labor). That said, there's a difference between old wives' tales (or what some think of as "folk wisdom") and what we're able to prove: a 2006 research study published in *Obstetrics &*

Gynecology found that sexual intercourse wasn't linked to going into labor.[10] Of course, if your health care provider has greenlighted sex for you and your partner, and you feel comfortable enough to have sex, then by all means go for it (gently) and see whether it works for you. You might want to leave those details out of the baby announcements, though!

SEX AFTER BABY

S ex during pregnancy is one thing; sex after pregnancy is a whole new ballgame. In a study published in the *British Journal of Obstetrics and Gynaecology*, researchers followed 119 women who were pregnant with their first child through their pregnancy and the year following delivery.[11] They found that by six weeks postpartum most of these first-time mothers had not resumed sexual intercourse—in fact, only about one-third reported doing so. However, the vast majority of women had done so by three months postpartum. Of course, that doesn't mean that sex was "the same" for them as it was before they were pregnant or had their baby. At three months postpartum, about three-quarters of women in the study reported less frequent intercourse compared to the month before they became pregnant. Even at twelve months postpartum, more than half of the women—57 percent—were having less frequent sex than before pregnancy.

That said, it may be that comparing sex post-baby with sex pre-pregnancy isn't the best comparison. After all, couples who are trying to conceive often have more sex than usual in an attempt to become pregnant, so the comparison with how frequent sex was before becoming pregnancy may not be ideal. For me, the biggest take-home message of this study is that just as children learn to walk and talk when they're ready, women who have recently had a baby readjust to sexual activity when they are ready too. The idea that many women can resume intercourse at six weeks after delivery is largely for health reasons. By no means does it mean that all women will be rested enough for enjoyable sex or that they will have sufficient desire by then (or that any genital pain will have subsided). Every pregnancy and birth experience is individual, as is every woman's relationship.

If you and your partner are struggling over this issue, I would encourage you to connect with a support and education group for new parents. Figuring out sex after baby is easy for some couples and challenging for others. Given the many new stresses that come with raising a baby (for example, sleep, breastfeeding, deciding whose turn it is to change a diaper), it's no wonder that sexuality, intimacy, and relationships change. Talking about it with your partner, trying to be patient, getting good-quality sleep so you feel rested enough to manage your relationship's ups and downs with grace, and a dose of humor will help.

— Making It Easy —

87. What to do if . . . you're in the third trimester and want to have sex, but aren't sure which positions are safe or risky

As long as your health care provider has given you the go-ahead to have sex as usual, then the sex position you choose is really up to you and your partner to decide on. There is no one "best" sex position, even in a woman's third trimester of pregnancy. A few studies have found that there may be a slight risk of preterm labor among women who have face-to-face missionary-style sex (with her male partner on top); however, other studies haven't found such a connection. In fact, a study published in a 2010 issue of the *Journal of Sexual and Marital Therapy* found that man-on-top missionary remains the most common sex position reported by pregnant women.[12] Not that there aren't others: the same study also found that more women who were highly sexually satisfied tended to opt for sex positions like woman on top, face-to-face sex, and positions that supported their growing bumps. Again, as long as your health care provider has deemed you good to go for sex during pregnancy, the sex position choice is largely yours—and it's no surprise that comfort matters. After all, if you can't relax and enjoy it, what's the point?

88. What to do if . . . you're distracted mid-sex by the baby monitor

If your baby is generally healthy, it's OK to turn the baby monitor off for a few minutes. You simply cannot hear your baby perfectly all of the time. Even if you take the monitor into the bathroom with you while you shower (I know: when do new moms and dads even seem to find the time for a decent shower?), you have to admit that it sounds a bit muffled with the shower wooshing by you. If you can reassure yourself that it's OK to turn the monitor off for a few minutes, you may be better suited to relax, let go, and enjoy sex. Turning your attention away from your baby and toward yourself and your partner can be good for your relationship—and thus good for the whole family.

If you feel truly concerned that your baby needs to be attended to, try to find other ways to focus on your relationship and make time to make love. You might hire a babysitter to take your baby on an hour-long walk while you and your partner stay at home together on a weekend afternoon. Or drop your baby off at her or his grandparents' house for a few hours while you make time for yourselves (and that shower).

89. What to do if . . . sex doesn't feel the same post-childbirth

Although labor and delivery are often over in a matter of hours, your sex life is likely to take a matter of months to feel close to normal again. While many health care providers give women and their partners the go-ahead to resume sexual activity four to six weeks after delivery, not all women feel ready to get back into sex that soon. For many women, it can take up to six months (or longer—even up to a year) to get back into the swing of sex. This can be for any number of reasons. Many women experience vaginal or perianal tearing during delivery. And while routine episiotomies are largely out of favor, some health care providers still perform them even when women, as part of their birth plans, specifically ask for an episiotomy to be avoided unless necessary. Consequently, women may experience sensitivity or pain in the area where their episiotomy scars are, or else they may experience other types of genital pain or discomfort following childbirth. If you're breastfeeding, you may be experiencing vaginal dryness due to low estrogen; using a vaginal lubricant and/or moisturizer can be helpful. Another common cause of sexual difficulties in the postpartum period has to do with lack of sleep: new parents are often exhausted, sleeping only for minutes or a few hours a time. In these cases, it is perfectly normal to put sex on the back burner so you can take care of yourselves.

Sex can change in varied ways. Some women find that certain go-to sex positions no longer produce pleasure or lead to orgasms for them. With encouragement, they often try other sex positions (including ones that used to do nothing for them) and sometimes—much to their pleasant surprise—they learn that their body now responds positively, and with pleasure and sometimes orgasm, to these new sex positions. In other words, post-childbirth changes to sex aren't always negative ones. Sometimes, they're good ones.

Many women find that it's helpful to connect with other new moms in support groups (ask your OB/GYN, local birth center, or midwife group for information about groups near you). These groups can be helpful for a number of reasons, from commiserating about a lack of sleep to getting advice on breastfeeding and even talking about changes related to sexual desire, positions, pleasure, pain, and orgasm. If you start talking about sex with other new moms, you're likely to open the flood gates to conversation.

90. What to do if . . . you want to masturbate two weeks after a C-section but aren't sure if it's okay

Some women feel ready to masturbate or have sex soon after giving birth, whether by C-section or vaginally. However, health care providers often recommend waiting four to six weeks following delivery (regardless of how you delivered) before resuming sex. And while they often just say "sex," this typically includes masturbation. Women who have had a C-section have had an incision in the uterus, which can take time to heal. It's also common to experience bleeding in the weeks following delivery. If you have questions about your own sex or masturbation timeline after delivery, ask your health care provider. Every woman, every pregnancy, and every new mom is different, so you'll get the most personally relevant information from your provider.

91. What to do if . . . you want to use a vibrator but worry that your roommate or neighbor will hear through the very thin walls

A number of vibrator characteristics matter to women and men. They often want toys that are affordable, easy to clean, high quality—and not terribly loud. It's not that people are worried about vibrators being so loud that they'll pierce their eardrums. Most vibrators aren't all that loud in comparison to other sounds in our homes or other environments. Rather, people often prefer relatively quiet vibrators so that nearby neighbors, housemates, parents, kids, or even pets won't hear the noise and be curious about what's going on. However, quiet vibrators tend to lack intensity. If you want a powerful, intense vibrator, you have to learn to deal with the sound its motor makes. No worries—if you need to drown your vibrator sound, try the following:

• **Choose a vibrator with a multispeed dial.** That way, you can lower the vibrator to a setting that meets a good middle ground of sound and intensity.

• **Masturbate under the covers,** with a thick comforter on top of you (and the vibrator).

• **Grab a pillow or two** and place it over the covers that are already over your hands and vibrator.

• **Play music.** As long as people have had record players or boom boxes in their rooms, they've been masking sex noises—including sex toy noises. Create a sex playlist (see my book, *Great in Bed,* for tips on how to do this) and use it when things get fun.

92. What to do if . . . your partner is recovering from surgery and you're not sure what you can or cannot do, sexually

If you or your partner has had recent surgery, ask the surgeon how quickly you can resume masturbation and/or sex together. Doctors rarely talk to patients about how surgery and other medical treatments may affect their sex lives, so it may be up to you to ask the initial question.

Get specific too. Ask what changes, if any, you will need to make to your sex life once you resume having sex. If you've had surgery for carpal tunnel syndrome, it may be some time before your surgeon thinks it's okay to use a vibrator. If you've had a knee replacement, there may be some sex positions (such as those that involve certain angles for, or pressure on, your knees) that are ill advised. If your surgeon seems uncomfortable answering sex-specific questions (most doctors have had very little, if any, training in sexual matters), then ask if there is anything specific you should avoid doing with your body—for example, ways you shouldn't use the part you had surgery on, and for how long. That may help you figure out what tweaks you need to make to your sex life. If you're seeing a physical therapist as part of your recovery, you may be able to ask him or her for additional tips about modifications to your sex life. Often, physical therapists get a sense from surgeons and doctors how patients' bodies should and shouldn't be moved post-surgery. Your physical therapist may be able to take that information and help translate it into sex tips that work for you.

Teaching the Birds and the Bees

Most parents I encounter want to give their children helpful, accurate, and developmentally appropriate information about their bodies and about how babies are made. This is good because these conversations help create comfortable opportunities for parents and their children to start talking about sexuality and reproduction in ways that are appropriate for children. Over time, children may notice that they can talk openly and comfortably with their parents. As they grow older, this is particularly helpful because it means they may be more likely to feel comfortable asking more advanced sex questions of their parents. For a good beginning, I recommend two books that parents can read to their young children. The first is called *It's Not the Stork!: A Book about Girls, Boys, Babies, Bodies,*

Families, and Friends. The second is *It's So Amazing! A Book about Eggs, Sperm, Birth, Babies, and Families*. Both are by Robie H. Harris and Michael Emberley.

93. What to do if . . . your child walks in on you having sex

If your child is very young (say, two or three years old), it's unlikely that they will remember any of this. And because your child is so young, you may have just as many questions for your child ("How did you get out of your crib?") as he or she has for you ("What are you doing?"). At such a young age, a common parental response is to reassure their child that the parent is OK (some young children are worried that pleasurable moans or orgasmic noises are signs of distress rather than joy) and see what it is the child needs (such as food, drink, or a diaper change).

Slightly older children may have more specific questions—and can understand more accurate answers. If a five- or six-year-old child walks in on their parents having sex, some parents ask their child to leave, and then they dress, join their child in another room, and explain what it is they saw (saying, for example, "Adults sometimes have sex with each other as a way of showing how much they like or love each other"). Other parents are more vague with their explanations. If you're raising a child, then whether your child is six months, six years, or sixteen years old, I highly recommend reading *From Diapers to Dating: A Parent's Guide to Raising Sexually Healthy Children* and/or *What Every 21st-Century Parent Needs to Know: Facing Today's Challenges with Wisdom and Heart*, both by Debra Haffner.

Finally, rest assured that in my work teaching college students and writing sex columns, I have yet to come across someone who feels they were truly traumatized by walking in to find their parents having sex. More often, these stories are funny and involve some level of discomfort, on both the child's and their parents' part, but they are not typically upsetting encounters. Often, children don't pay much attention to the episode until years later when they have a more advanced understanding of what sex is and then look back and realize what they witnessed when they were younger.

94. What to do if . . . your cat shows more interest in your toys than her own

Sex toys and cats don't mix. Several women have told me that their cats are curious about their vibrators and even bat them around with their paws (cats do love moving objects, whether it's string or a cat toy dragged along the carpet . . . I guess vibrators aren't that different). When you're using your vibrator, try to keep your cat busy in another room, such as with catnip, its meal, or a toy of its own. When you're not using your vibrator, catproof it by locking it away in a box or a nightstand drawer—someplace where your cat is unlikely to find it. Lubricant, too, should be kept with the cap on and somewhere out of your cat's reach, as it's probably not good for them.

Our cat likes our lubricant. We always have to make sure it's covered.
—Dan, age fifty-one

95. What to do if . . . your dog barks when you and your partner try to kiss or cuddle

In my "pets and sex" study, it was a common occurrence for dogs to get feisty as their "dog parents" got kissy or huggy. About one in five dog owners and close to 10 percent of cat owners said that their pet sometimes or often interfered with their hugging. Similar numbers reported pet interruptions when they and their partner kissed. Cuddling was particularly tricky: close to 30 percent of dog and cat owners reported that their pet sometimes or often interfered with their cuddling attempts. Because recent research from a colleague at the Kinsey Institute found that touching, cuddling, and kissing play an important part in men's sexual satisfaction (and let's face it, most of us like a good cuddle), it's worth figuring out how to balance this part of your life so you can enjoy your pets and enjoy your partner too.

Our dog, Jezebel, barks when we stand and hug and kiss one another hello or good-bye. Sometimes we keep up with it anyway, barking be damned. Other times we put her in a "down" position to quiet her. Still other times, we simply turn to the side, open our arms, and invite her to join our "hug circle" after she's been quiet for a moment; she then stands on her hind legs and puts her paws on us to join the hug. Other people put their pets in another room if they're down for some serious cuddle time. Some people give their dogs peanut butter–filled dog toys or throw some catnip their cats' way. You know your pet best; to the extent that you can create some touchy-feely space for you and your partner, it can be a good part of your relationship.

96. What to do if . . . you're starting to get sexually serious with someone who has a pet—and you have an allergy

It depends how serious your allergy is. Some people have one or more pet-free rooms in their home (that the pet is never allowed to enter, including when the person isn't there) to accommodate an allergic partner. Often, one of these pet-free rooms is the bedroom, which can make for an easier time sexually. Other times, the nonallergic pet owner makes the trip to the allergic partner's place when they want to get naked. It can help for the pet owner to put on clean clothes that are free of pet hair before they visit their allergic partner. It may also help if the person with the pet refrains from kissing their pet good-bye before leaving, lest their lips end up having traces of dog or cat that may rub off later, via a kiss or oral sex, on their partner.

If a person has a severe allergy to dogs or cats, he or she may decide that it's best to avoid dating pet owners. It may narrow one's dating pool, but it's important to take care of one's health. If you have any questions about steps you should take to deal with your allergies, consult a health care provider, such as an allergy specialist.

97. What to do if . . . you're too tired for sex because your cat or dog wakes you up night after night

We may not talk openly about it, but new parents, people with sleep apnea, and overworked individuals aren't the only ones who suffer from sleep disturbance. Pet owners are often struck with sleep difficulties too. A Mayo Clinic study found that a sizable number of its sleep disorder patients let their pets sleep with them. In another study, Austrian researchers used a device worn around a person's wrist during sleep to discover that people experienced greater sleep difficulties when their dog slept in the same bed as them than when their dog slept elsewhere. And in my post-pet sex study, I found that about a third of dog and cat owners typically slept with their pet in the bed. Of those who shared the bed with their pet, about a quarter of dog owners and 12 percent of cat owners said their pet slept between them and their partner. And nearly half of dog and cat owners said their pet woke them up at least once during a typical night. Given how important sleep is to feeling rested, energetic, relaxed, and happy—not to mention avoiding accidents on the road—we should all perhaps find ways to experience sounder sleep.

There are a number of steps you can take to improve your sleep life (and better sleep can set you up for better sex). Try to support your natural sleep rhythms by using bright lights during the day and dimmer lights in the evening. If possible, limit your exposure to bright screens (like televisions and laptops) in the hour before you normally go to sleep. Keeping to a regular sleep schedule can help too, as can sleeping in a dark room with dark shades. And as far as your pets are concerned, if your dog is a puppy, it's a prime time to crate train them so that they will learn to sleep in a crate rather than your bed. Not into the crate idea? That's OK: you can still train them to sleep in another room or in their own dog bed rather than in your bed. Cats, too, can be trained to sleep elsewhere, particularly if their water, litter box, and food bowl are there too.

Of course, some people really enjoy having their pet to cuddle with, and that should be respected too. It can feel meaningful and loving to share one's bed with a pet. And for some people, sharing their bed with both their partner and a pet brings the two people closer as they cuddle together with their pet and laugh about the silly things it does (like burrow under the covers or pounce on their feet).

The dog is crated at night, so it's no problem for nighttime sex. For daytime sex or spontaneous sex, we will usually shut the door to our bedroom or crate the dog if we are having sex outside the bedroom. Sometimes we will put her outside because she thinks that playful wrestling and teasing for foreplay is a game that she wants to be part of (and, obviously, a cold wet

nose or sharp toenail at the wrong moment can derail the fore-
play for a bit).
—Anna, age twenty-six

98. What to do if . . . you'd love to spoon with your partner at night if only your pet didn't crawl into bed between you two

Either find a new place for your pet to sleep aside from the bed (see above) or see if you can relocate your pet to sleep by your feet. Some people can be very sensitive about any attempt to move their pet's place of sleep. I know some men and women who adore sleeping with their pets and have ended relationships with partners who wanted the pet to sleep elsewhere, so you may need to proceed delicately. Try to frame it in terms of a positive for your partner by saying something like

> *"I'd really like to be closer to you at night, to be able to cuddle and spoon, but the dog/cat is often between us. Can you brainstorm with me to figure out how we can get a little closer?"*

> *"When we sleep close together, it turns me on to feel your body right up against mine, but sometimes I wake up and find I'm spooning the dog/cat instead of you. What do you think about training the dog/cat to sleep elsewhere?"*

Training a pet to sleep elsewhere can take time, patience, and consistency. If you truly don't want your pet to sleep with you, keep your pet out of the bed night after night. Letting him or her in the bed some nights but not others can be confusing for the pet. Seek help from an animal behavior specialist or a trainer if you have questions about effective training techniques.

> *The cats pretty much do what they please while we are having sex. Usually, they jump off the bed because we are disturbing them. Sometimes, we will notice one of them watching, and it's a little odd, but not that big of a deal. The main disturbance that*

the cats have for us during sex is when they pounce on our feet under the covers. We usually laugh about it and keep going.
—Lana, age twenty-six

99. What to do if . . . you feel like your cat is getting in the way of your dating life because you have to come home in the morning to feed him or her

If your cat isn't a food-ravenous monster and instead only eats in moderation, you may be able to get away with leaving a large amount of food out. If, instead, your cat eats everything in sight right away, using a food timing device may work better. One woman in my post-pet sex study said that she found a "food ball" to be effective for nights when she sleeps over at her partner's house. A food ball is a toy-like product that a cat has to persistently work at to get the food to release, meaning it takes time (and a lot of playfulness) to do. Food balls often have small holes in them. You fill them with dry food and then, as your cat chases the ball around, the dry food escapes the hole little by little, giving you more time to sleep in with your partner. Of course, an alternative is to ask your partner to sleep over at your place so you can give your cat breakfast in the morning.

100. What to do if . . . you're distracted during sex by your dog's stares

Again, it all goes back to where you've trained your dog to hang out and how well trained your dog is. If your dog can get into a "down stay" position on command, then even if you have a one-room studio apartment you can ask your dog to lie down facing away from you so you can have sex without seeing any stares. You might even turn the lights out so as not to make eye contact with an awkwardly staring pooch. Another option is to simply not look in his or her direction, no matter what you do. In my post-pet sex study, some said that their dog crawls under the bed when they have sex. However, one woman said this stressed her out because she worried that the bed would collapse one day during sex and hurt her dog. Of course, you can also just laugh about it: sex is full of surprises and occasional awkward moments, and a little awkward dog staring may be par for the sex course.

Sex Smarts Quiz

1. If a person feels that they are practically "watching themselves" have sex and criticizing themselves or worrying about their performance, this may be an example of
    a. Tenting
    b. Spectatoring
    c. Arousal
    d. Body image concerns
2. True or false: Most women are able to have sex through out pregnancy.
3. About how many pet owners allow their pet to sleep in their bed?
    a. 5 percent
    b. 10 percent
    c. 33 percent
    d. 75 percent

Answers
    1. b
    2. True
    3. c

Resources

Books

Boston Women's Health Book Collective. (2005). *Our Bodies, Ourselves: A New Edition for a New Era.* New York: Simon & Schuster.

Boston Women's Health Book Collective. (2008). *Our Bodies, Ourselves: Pregnancy and Birth.* New York: Touchstone Book/Simon & Schuster.

Boston Women's Health Book Collective. (2006). *Our Bodies, Ourselves: Menopause.* New York: Simon & Schuster.

Dodson, B. (1996). *Sex for One: The Joy of Selfloving.* New York: Crown Trade Paperbacks.

Dodson, B. (2002). *Orgasms for Two: The Joy of Partnersex.* New York: Harmony.

Ensler, E. (2001). *The Vagina Monologues.* New York: Villard.

Heiman, J., & J. LoPiccolo, (1988). *Becoming Orgasmic: A Sexual and Personal Growth Program for Women.* New York: Prentice Hall.

Herbenick, D. (2009). *Because It Feels Good: A Woman's Guide to Sexual Pleasure and Satisfaction.* Emmaus, PA: Rodale.

Herbenick, D. (2011). *The Good in Bed Guide to Anal Pleasuring.* New York: Good in Bed Guides. (Digital e-book).

Herbenick, D. and V. Schick, (2011). *Read My Lips: A Complete Guide to the Vagina and Vulva.* Lanham, MD: Rowman & Littlefield.

Komisaruk, B. R., C. Beyer, & B. Whipple, (2006). *The Science of Orgasm.* Baltimore: Johns Hopkins University Press.

Redd, N. A. (2007). *Body drama*. New York: Gotham Books.

Schnarch, D. *Passionate Marriage: Keeping Love and Intimacy Alive in Committed Relationships*. New York: W. W. Norton & Company.

Stewart, E. G. & P. Spencer (2002). *The V book: A Doctor's Guide to Complete Vulvovaginal Health*. New York: Bantam Books.

Organizations

American Association of Sexuality Educators, Counselors and Therapists (AASECT)
1444 I Street NW, Suite 700, Washington, DC 20005
Web: www.aasect.org
Phone: 202.449.1099
Offers educational materials and the ability to search for sex counselors and therapists in your area.

American Congress of Obstetricians and Gynecologists
PO Box 96920, Washington, DC 20090-6920
Web: www.acog.org
Phone: 202.638.5577
Patient brochures and information materials are available online.

American Psychological Association
750 First Street NE, Washington, DC 20002-4242
Web: www.apa.org
Phone: 800.374.2721
Offers educational materials and the ability to search for providers in your area.

American Social Health Association (ASHA)
P.O. Box 13827, Research Triangle Park, NC 27709
Web: www.ashastd.org
Phone: 919.361.8400
Provides a wealth of information about sexually transmissible infections
(STIs).

The International Society for the Study of Vulvovaginal Disease
(ISSVD)
8814 Peppergrass Lane, Waxhaw, NC 28173
Web: www.issvd.org
Phone: 704.814.9493
Patient information materials are available; you can also contact the ISSVD
to request information about finding vulvovaginal health care specialists
in your area.

Planned Parenthood
434 W. 33rd Street, New York, NY 10001
Web: www.plannedparenthood.org
Phone: 800.230.PLAN (7526)
Health information is available online including information related to STIs,
birth control, gynecological health care, and abortion services.

National Vulvodynia Association
PO Box 4491, Silver Spring, MD 20914-4491
Web: www.nva.org
Phone: 301.299.0755 (3999: fax)
Information and resources related to vulvar pain.

Society for Sex Therapy and Research
6311 W. Gross Point Rd., Niles, IL 60714
Web: www.sstarnet.org
Phone: 847.647.8832
Find a sex therapist in your area.

The Kinsey Institute

Morrison Hall 302, 1165 E. Third St., Bloomington, IN 47405 USA

Web: www.kinseyinstitute.org and www.kinseyconfidential.org

Phone: 812.855.7686

Information and resources related to sexuality. Also, the Kinsey Confidential service provides answers to commonly asked questions about sex (answered by Dr. Debby Herbenick) as does the Kinsey Confidential podcast series, which is available for free download.

The New View Campaign

POB 1845, New York, NY 10159-1845

Web: www.newviewcampaign.org

Provides information about the medicalization of women's sexuality and opportunities for activism.

Sex Shops and Boutiques

Babeland

www.babeland.com

800.658.9119

Early to Bed

www.early2bed.com

866.585.2BED (2233)

Good Vibrations

www.goodvibes.com

800.BUY.VIBE

My Pleasure

www.mypleasure.com

866.697.5327

Passion Parties
www.passionparties.com
800.4.PASSION

Pure Romance
www.pureromance.com
1.866.ROMANCE

Self Serve Toys
www.selfservetoys.com
505.265.5815

Smitten Kitten
www.smittenkittenonline.com
888.751.0523

Tulip Toy Gallery
www.mytulip.com
877.70.TULIP

Endnotes

Chapter 1

1. Handler, C. (2010). *Chelsea Chelsea Bang Bang*. Grand Central Publishing. New York, NY.

2. Mallants, C. and Casteels, K. (2008). Practical approach to childhood masturbation – a review. *European Journal of Pediatrics*, 167(10): 1111-1117.

3. Lawhead, R.A. and Majmudar, B. (1990). Early diagnosis of vulvar neoplasia as a result of vulvar self-examination. *Journal of Reproductive Medicine*, 35(12), 1134-1137.

4. Herbenick, D., Schick, V., Reece, M., Sanders, S.A., & Fortenberry, J.D. (2010). Pubic hair removal among women in the United States: prevalence, methods and characteristics. *Journal of Sexual Medicine*, 7, 3322-3330.

5. Tiggemann, M. and Hodgson, S. (2008). The hairlessness norm extended: reasons for and predictors of women's body hair removal at different body sites. *Sex Roles*, 59(11-12), 889-897.

6. Levin, R. (2003). The ins and outs of vaginal lubrication. *Sexual and Relationship Therapy*, 18(4), 509-513.

7. Hines, TM. (2001). The G-spot: a modern gynecologic myth. *American Journal of Obstetrics and Gynecology*, 185(2): 359-362.

8. Gravina, G.L., Brandetti, F., Martini, P., Carosa, E., Stasi, S.M., Morano, S., Lenzi, A., and Jannini, E.A. (2008). Measurement of the thickness of the urethrovaginal space in women with or without vaginal orgasm. *Journal of Sexual Medicine*, 5(3): 610-618.

9. Burri, A.V., Cherkas, L. and Spector, T.D. (2010). Genetic and environmental influences on self-reported G-Spots in women: a twin study. *Journal of Sexual Medicine*, 7(5): 1842-1852.

10. Herbenick, D., Reece, M., Schick, V., Sanders, S.A., Dodge, B., & Fortenberry, J.D. (2010). An event-level analysis of the sexual characteristics and composition among adults ages 18 to 59: results from a national probability sample in the United States. *Journal of Sexual Medicine*, 7 (suppl 5), 346-361.

11. Reitsma, W., Mourits, M.J.E., Koning, M., Pascal, A., and van der Lei, B. (2011). No (wo)man is an island- the influence of physicians' personal predisposition to labia minora appearance on their clinical decision making: a cross-sectional survey. *Journal of Sexual Medicine*, 8(8): 2377-2385.

12. Leiblum, S. and Nathan, S.G. (2001). Persistent sexual arousal syndrome: a newly discovered pattern of female sexuality. *Journal of Sex & Marital Therapy*, 27(4): 365-380.

13. Amsterdam, A., Abu-Rustum, N., Carter, J. and Krychman, M. (2005). Persistent sexual arousal syndrome associated with increased soy intake. *Journal of Sexual Medicine*, 2(3), 338-340.

14. Leiblum, S., Seehuus, M., Goldmeier, D., Brown, C. (2007). Psychological, medical and pharmacological correlates of persistent genital arousal disorder. *Journal of Sexual Medicine*, 4(5): 1358-1366.

15. Herbenick, D., Reece, M., Schick, V., Sanders, S.A., Dodge, B., & Fortenberry, J.D. (2010). An event-level analysis of the sexual characteristics and composition among adults ages 18 to 59: results from a national probability sample in the United States. *Journal of Sexual Medicine*, 7 (suppl 5), 346-361.

16. Zaviacic, M., Dolezalova, S., Holoman, I.K., Zaviacicova, A., Mikulecky, M., & Brazdil, V. (1998). Concentrations of fructose in female ejaculate and urine: a comparative biochemical study. *Journal of Sex Research*, 24(1): 319-325.

17. Addiego, F., Belzer, E.G., Comolli, J., Moger, W., Perry, J.D., and Whipple, B. (1981). Female ejaculation: a case study. *Journal of Sex Research*, 17(1): 13-21.

Chapter 2

1. Kinsey AC, Pomery WB, Martin CE. *Sexual Behavior in the Human Male*. Philadelphia, PA: W. B. Saunders Company; 1948.

2. Lever, J. and Frederick, D.A. (2006). Does size matter? Men's and women's views on penis size across the lifespan. *Psychology of Men & Masculinity*, 7(3), 129-143.

3. Male circumcision: Global trends and determinants of prevalence, safety and acceptability" (PDF). World Health Organization. 2007. http://whqlibdoc.who.int/publications/2007/9789241596169_eng.pdf. Retrieved October 10, 2011.

4. Lavreys, L., Rakwar, J.P., Thompson, M.L., Jackson, D.J., Mandaliya, K., Choban, B.H., Bwayo, J.J., Ndinya-Achola, J.O., and Kreiss, J.K. (1999). Effect of circumcision on incident of human immunodeficiency virus Type 1 and other sexually transmitted diseases: a prospective cohort study of trucking company employees in Kenya. *Journal of Infectious Disease*, 180(2), 330-336.

5. Millett, G.A., Flores, S.A., Marks, G., Reed, J.B., Herbst, J.H. (2008). Circumcision status and risk of HIV and sexually transmitted infections among men who have sex with men. *Journal of the American Medical Association*, 300(14): 1674-1684.

6. O'Hara, K. and O'Hara, J. (1999). The effect of male circumcision on the sexual enjoyment of the female partner. *British Journal of Urology*, 83(S1): 79-84.

7. Richters, J., Gerofi, J. and Donovan, B. (1995). Why do condoms break or slip off in use? An exploratory study. International *Journal of STD and AIDS*, 6(1): 11-18.

8. Leitzmann, M.F., Platz, E.A., Stampfer, M.J., Willett, W.C., and Giovannucci, E. (2004). Ejaculation frequency and subsequent risk of prostate cancer. *Journal of the American Medical Association*, 291(13): 1578-1586.

9. Herbenick, D., Reece, M., Sanders, S.A., Dodge, B., Ghassemi, A., & Fortenberry, J.D. (2009). Prevalence and characteristics of vibrator use by women in the United States: Results from a nationally representative study. *Journal of Sexual Medicine*, 6, 1857-1866.

10. Kramer, A.C. (2011). Penile fracture seems more likely during sex under stressful situations. *Journal of Sexual Medicine*. Published online ahead of print. DOI: 10.1111/j.1743-6109.2011.02461.x

11. Armstrong, M.L., Caliendo, C., and Roberts, A.E. (2006). Genital piercings: what is known and what people with genital piercings tell us. *Urologic Nursing*, 26(2): 176-179.

12. Lee-Wong, M., Collins, J.S., Cyrus, N., and Resnick, D.J. (2008). Diagnosis and treatment of human seminal plasma hypersensitivity. *Obstetrics & Gynecology*, 111(2): 538-539.

13. Ludman, B.G. (1999). Human seminal plasma protein allergy: a diagnosis rarely considered. *Journal of Obstetric, Gynecologic & Neonatal Nursing*, 28(4), 359-363.

14. Zukerman, Z., Weiss, D.B., and Orvieto, R. (2003). Does pre-ejaculatory penile secretion originating from Cowper's gland contain sperm? *Journal of Assisted Reproduction and Genetics*, 20(4): 157-159.

15. Jones, R.K., Fennell, J., Higgins, J.A., and Blanchard, K. (2009). Better than nothing or savvy risk-reduction practice? The importance of withdrawal. *Contraception*, 79(6), 407-410.

16. Niederberger, C.S. and Chudnovsky, A. (2007). Copious pre-ejaculation: small glands – major headaches. *Journal of Andrology*, 28(3): 374-375.

Chapter 3

1. Hensel, D. J., Stupiansky, N.W., Herbenick, D., Dodge, B., & Reece, M. (2011). When condom use is not condom use: an event-level analysis of condom use behaviors during vaginal intercourse. *Journal of Sexual Medicine*, 8(1), 28-34.

2. Stone, N., Hatherall, B., Ingham, R., and McEachran, J. (2006). Oral sex and condom use among young people in the United Kingdom. *Perspectives on Sexual and Reproductive Health*, 38(1): 6-12.

3. Dunne, E.F., Unger, E.R., Sternberg, M., McQuillan, G., Swan, D.C., Patel, S.S., and Markowitz, L.E. (2007). Prevalence of HPV infection among females in the United States. *Journal of the American Medical Association*, 297(8): 813-819.

4. Centers for Disease Control and Prevention. Genital Herpes – CDC Fact Sheet. Retrieved on October 10, 2011 from: http://cdc.gov/std/Herpes/STDFact-Herpes.htm

5. Pitt, S., Boyinton, C., Sutherland, K., Lovgren, M., Tilley, P., Read, R., and Singh, A.E. (2009). Antimicrobial resistance in gonorrhea: the influence of epidemiologic and laboratory surveillance data on treatment guidelines: Alberta, Canada 2001-2007. *Sexually Transmitted Diseases*, 36(10): 656-669.

6. Barry, P.M. and Klausner, J.D. (2009). The use of cephalosporins for gonorrhea: the impending problem of resistance. *Expert Opinion on Pharmacotherapy*, 10(4): 555-577.

7. Fortenberry, J.D., Schick, V., Herbenick, D., Sanders, S.A., Dodge, B., & Reece, M. (2010). Sexual behaviors and condom use at last vaginal intercourse: a national sample of adolescents ages 14 to 17 years. *Journal of Sexual Medicine*, 7 (suppl 5), 305-314.

8. Marur, S., D'Souza, G., Westra, W.H., and Forastiere, A.A. (2010). HPV-associated head and neck cancer: a virus-related cancer epidemic. *The Lancet Oncology*, 11(8): 781-789.

9. Coutant-Foulc, P., Lewis, F., Berville, S., Guihard, P., Renaut, J.J., Reid, W., and Barracco, M.M. (2011). Unilateral vulvar swelling as a consequence of intensive cycling: report of 5 cases. *Journal of Lower Genital Tract Disease*, Supplement S8.

10. Goldstein, I., Lurie, A.L., and Lubisich, J.P. (2007). Bicycle riding, perineal trauma, and erectile dysfunction: data and solutions. *Current Urology Reports*, 8(6): 491-497.

Chapter 4

1. Wellings, K., Field, J., Johnson, A., Wadsworth, J. (eds). *Sexual Behavior in Britain*. London. Penguin Books, 1994: 265.

2. Heiman, J., Long, S., Smith, S.N., Fisher, W.A., Sand, M.S., and Rosen, R.C. (2011). Sexual satisfaction and relationship happiness in midlife and older couples in five countries. *Archives of Sexual Behavior*, 40, 741–753.

3. Wallen, K. and Lloyd, E. (2011). Female sexual arousal: genital anatomy and orgasm in intercourse. *Hormones and Behavior*, 59(5): 780-792.

4. Herbenick, D., Reece, M., Schick, V., Sanders, S.A., Dodge, B., & Fortenberry, J.D. (2010). An event-level analysis of the sexual characteristics and composition among adults ages 18 to 59: results from a national probability sample in the United States. *Journal of Sexual Medicine*, 7 (suppl 5), 346-361.

5. Holstege, G. and Huynh, H.K. (2011). Brain circuits for mating behavior in cats and brain activations and de-activations during sexual stimulation and ejaculation and orgasm in humans. *Hormones and Behavior*, 59(5): 702-707.

6. Komisaruk, B.R., Wise, N., Frangos, E., Liu, W.C., Allen, K., and Brody, S. (2011). Women's clitoris, vagina and cervix mapped on the sensory cortex: fMRI evidence. *Journal of Sexual Medicine*, 8(10), 2822-2830.

7. Saha, P. (2002). Breastfeeding and sexuality: professional advice literature from the 1970s to the present. *Health Education and Behavior*, 29(1), 61-72.

8. Frese, A., Eikermann, A., Frese, K., Schwaag, S., Husstedt, I.W., and Evers, S. (2003). Headache associated with sexual activity: demography, clinical features and comorbidity. *Neurology*, 61(6): 796-800.

9. Nurnberg, H.G., Hensley, P.L., Heiman, J.R., Croft, H.A., Debattista, C., & Paine, S. (2008). Sildenafil Treatment of Women With Antidepressant-Associated Sexual Dysfunction. *Journal of the American Medical Association*, 300(4): 395-404.

10. Dragisic, K.G. and Milad, M.P. (2004). Sexual functioning and patient expectations of sexual functioning after hysterectomy. *American Journal of Obstetrics and Gynecology*, 190(5), 1416-1418.

Chapter 5

1. Kubin, M., Wagner, G., and Fugl-Meyer, A.R. (2003). Epidemiology of erectile dysfunction. *International Journal of Impotence Research*, 15, 63-71.

2. Jern, P., Santtila, P., Witting, K., Alanko, K., Harlaar, N., Johansson, A., Von Der Pahlen, B., Varjonen, M., Vikstrom, N., Algars, M., and Sandnabba, K. (2007). Premature and delayed ejaculation: genetic and environ-mental effects in a population-based sample of Finnish twins. *Journal of Sexual Medicine*, 4(6), 1739-1749.

3. Gupta, B.P., Murad, H., Clifton, M.M., Prokop, L., Nehra, A., and Kopecky, S.L. (2011). The effect of lifestyle modification and cardiovascular risk factor reduction on erectile dysfunction: a systematic review and meta-analysis. *Archives of Internal Medicine*, Published online ahead of print. doi:10.1001/archinternmed.2011.440

4. Levin, R. (2009). Revisiting post-ejaculation refractory time: what we know and what we do not know in males and in females. *Journal of Sexual Medicine*, 6(9): 2376-2389.

5. Zilbergeld, B. (1999). *The New Male Sexuality*. New York: Bantam.

6. Dhikav, V., Karmarkar, G., Gupta, M. and Anand, K.S. (2007). Yoga in premature ejaculation: a comparative trial with fluoxetine. *Journal of Sexual Medicine*, 4(6): 1726-1732

7. Althof, S.E., Abdo, C.H.N., Dean, J., Hackett, G., McCabe, M., McMahon, C.G., Rosen, R.C., Sadovsky, R., Waldinger, M., Becher, E., Broderick, G.A., Buvat, J., Goldstein, I., El-Meliegy, A.I., Giuliano, F., Hellstrom, W.J.G.,

8. Incrocci, L., Jannini, E.A., Park, K., Parish, S., Porst, H., Rowland, D., Segraves, R., Sharlip, I., Simonelli, C., and Tan, H.M. (2010). International Society for Sexual Medicine's guidelines for the diagnosis and treatment of premature ejaculation. *Journal of Sexual Medicine*, 7(9), 2947-2969.

9. Sanders, S.A., Milhausen, R.R., Crosby, R.A., Graham, C.A., and Yarber, W.L. (2009). Do phosphodiesterase type 5 inhibitors protect against condom-associated erection loss and condom slippage? *Journal of Sexual Medicine*, 6(5), 1451-1456.

10. Benninger, M.S., Khalid, A.N., Benninger, R.M. and Smith, T.L. (2010). Surgery for chronic rhinosinusitis may improve sleep and sexual function. *The Laryngoscope*, 120(8): 1696-1700.

Chapter 6

1. Butzer, B. and Campbell, L. (2008). Adult attachment, sexual satisfaction, and relationship satisfaction: a study of married couples. *Personal Relationships*, 15(1), 141-154.

2. Davies, S., Katz, J., and Jackson, J.L. (1999). Sexual desire discrepancies: effects on sexual and relationship satisfaction in heterosexual dating couples. *Archives of Sexual Behavior*, 28(6): 553-567.

3. Smith, C.V. (2007). In pursuit of 'good' sex: self-determination and the sexual experience. *Journal of Social and Personal Relationships*, 24(1), 69-85.

4. Weaver, A.D. and Byers, E.S. (2006). The relationships among body image, body mass index, exercise, and sexual functioning in heterosexual women. *Psychology of Women Quarterly*, 30(4), 333-339.

5. Satinsky, S., Reece, M., Dennis, B., Sanders, S., and Bardzell, S. An assessment of body appreciation and its relationship to sexual function in women. *Body Image*. Published online ahead of print on October 22, 2011. Doi:10.1016/j.bodyim.2011.09.007.

6. Aron, A., Steele, J.L., Kashdan, T.B., and Perez, M. (2006). When similars do not attract: tests of a prediction from the self-expansion model. *Personal Relationships*, 13(4), 387-396.

7. Aron, A., Norman, C.C., Aron, E.N., McKenna, C. and Heyman, R.E. (2000). Couples' shared participation in novel and arousing activities and experienced relationship quality. *Journal of Personality and Social Psychology*, 78(2), 273-284.

8. Ebrahim, I.O. (2006). Somnambulistic sexual behavior (sexsomnia). *Journal of Clinical Forensic Medicine*, 13(4), 219-224.

Chapter 7

1. Herbenick, D., Reece, M., Sanders, S.A., Dodge, B., Ghassemi, A., & Fortenberry, J.D. (2009). Prevalence and characteristics of vibrator use by women in the United States: Results from a nationally representative study. *Journal of Sexual Medicine*, 6, 1857-1866.

2. Reece, M., Herbenick, D., Sanders, S.A., Dodge, B., Ghassemi, A., & Fortenberry, J.D. (2009). Prevalence and characteristics of vibrator use by men in the United States. *Journal of Sexual Medicine*, 6, 1867-1874.

3. Dodson, B. (1996). *Sex for One: The Joy of Selfloving*. New York: Three Rivers Press.

4. Heiman, J. and LoPiccolo, J. (1988). *Becoming Orgasmic: A Sexual and Personal Growth Program for Women* New York: Fireside.

5. Herbenick, D., Reece, M., Sanders, S.A., Dodge, B., Ghassemi, A., & Fortenberry, J.D. (2010). Women's vibrator use in romantic relationships: Results from a nationally representative survey in the United States. *Journal of Sex & Marital Therapy*, 36, 49-65.

6. Herbenick, D., Reece, M., Schick, V., Jozkowski, K., Middlestadt, S., Sanders, S., Dodge, B., Ghassemi, A., & Fortenberry, J.D. (in press). Beliefs about women's vibrator use: results from a nationally representative survey in the United States. *Journal of Sex & Marital Therapy*, 37(5), 329-345.

Chapter 8

1. Herbenick, D., Reece, M., Sanders, S.A., Schick, V., Dodge, B., & Fortenberry, J.D. (2010). Sexual behavior in the United States: Results from a national probability sample of males and females ages 14 to 94. *Journal of Sexual Medicine*, 7 (suppl 5), 255-265.

2. Herbenick, D., Reece, M., Schick, V., Sanders, S.A., Dodge, B., & Fortenberry, J.D. (2010s). Sexual behaviors, relationships, and perceived health among adult women in the United States: Results from a national probability sample. *Journal of Sexual Medicine*, 7 (suppl 5), 277-290

3. Reece, M., Herbenick, D., Schick, V., Sanders, S.A., Dodge, B., & Fortenberry, J.D. (2010). Sexual behaviors, relationships, and perceived health among adult men in the United States: Results from a national probability sample. *Journal of Sexual Medicine*, 7 (suppl 5), 291-304.

4. Reece, M., Herbenick, D., Schick, V., Sanders, S.A.., Dodge, B., & Fortenberry, J.D. (2010). Condom use rates in a national probability sample of males and females ages 14 to 94 in the United States. *Journal of Sexual Medicine*, 7 (suppl 5), 266-276.

5. Herbenick, D., Reece, M., Schick, V., Sanders, S.A., Dodge, B., & Fortenberry, J.D. (2010). An event-level analysis of the sexual characteristics and composition among adults ages 18 to 59: results from a national probability sample in the United States. *Journal of Sexual Medicine*, 7 (suppl 5), 346-361.

6. Hicks, T.V. and Leitenberg, H. (2001). Sexual fantasies about one's partner versus someone else: gender differences in incidence and frequency. *Journal of Sex Research*, 38(1), 43-50.

Chapter 9

1. Meana, M. and Nunnick, S.E. (2006). Gender differences in the content of cognitive distraction during sex. *Journal of Sex Research*, 43(1), 59-67.

2. Lacefield, L. and Negy, C. Non-erotic cognitive distractions during sexual activity in sexual minority and heterosexual young adults. *Archives of Sexual Behavior*. Published online ahead of print, October 2011.

3. Brotto, L. and Heiman, J. (2007). Mindfulness in sex therapy: applications for women with sexual difficulties following gynecologic cancer. *Sexual & Relationship Therapy*, 22(1), 3-11.

4. Brotto, L.A., Krychman, M. and Jacobson, P. (2008). Eastern approaches for enhancing women's sexuality: mindfulness, acupuncture, and yoga (CME). *Journal of Sexual Medicine*, 5(12), 2741-2748.

5. *U.S. Pet Ownership & Demographics Sourcebook* (2007). A publication of the American Veterinary Medical Association.

6. Livingston, G. and Cohn. D. (2010). The new demography of American Motherhood. Pew Research Center. Revised August 19, 2010. Accessed online on October 15, 2011 from: http://pewresearch.org/pubs/1586/changing-demographic-characteristics-american-mothers

7. Naldoni, L.M.V., Pazmino, M.A.V., Pezzan, P.A.O., Pereira, S.B., Duarte, G. and Ferreira, C.H.J. (2011). Evaluation of sexual function in Brazilian pregnant women. *Journal of Sex & Marital Therapy*, 37(2), 116-129.

8. Pauls, R.N., Occhino, J.A., and Dryfhout, V.L. (2008). Effects of pregnancy on female sexual function and body image: a prospective study. *Journal of Sexual Medicine*, 5(8), 1915-1922.

9. Sagiv-Reiss, D.M., Birnbaum, G.E., and Safir, M.P. Changes in sexual experiences and relationship quality during pregnancy. *Archives of Sexual Behavior*. Published online ahead of print, October 2011. DOI: 10.1007/s10508-011-9839-9 Online First™

10. Schaffir, J. (2006). Sexual intercourse at term and onset of labor. *Obstetrics & Gynecology*, 107(6), 1310-1314.

11. Robson, K.M., Brant, H.A., and Kumar, R. (1981). Maternal sexuality during first pregnancy and after childbirth. *British Journal of Obstetrics & Gynaecology*, 88(9), 882-889.

12. Lee, J.T., Lin, C.L., Wan, G.H., and Liang, C.C. (2010). Sexual positions and sexual satisfaction of pregnant women. *Journal of Sex & Marital Therapy*, 36(5), 408-420.

Index